McGraw-Hill Clinical Care Plans

Pediatric Nursing

Notice

Medicine is an ever-changing science. As new research and clinical experience broaden our knowledge, changes in treatment and drug therapy are required. The editors and publisher of this work have checked with sources believed to be reliable in their efforts to provide information that is complete and generally in accord with the standards accepted at the time of publication. However, in view of the possibility of human error or changes in medical sciences, neither the editors nor the publisher nor any other party who has been involved in the preparation or publication of this work warrants that the information contained herein is in every respect accurate or complete, and they are not responsible for any errors or omissions or for the results obtained from the use of such information. Readers are encouraged to confirm the information contained herein with other sources. For example and in particular, readers are advised to check the product information sheet included in the package of each drug they plan to administer to be certain that the information contained in this book is accurate and that changes have not been made in the recommended dose or in the contraindications for administration. This recommendation is of particular importance in connection with new or infrequently used drugs.

To my mother, Joanne

CONTENTS

REVIEWERS AND CONTRIBUTORS

CLINICAL REVIEWERS

Bren Groves, RN, MN
Nurse Educator
Pediatric Critical Care

Nancy G. Hoyt, RN, MN
Director of Nursing
Medical/Surgical

Mary L. Krywanio, RN, DNS
Director
Nursing Education and Research

Denise LeBaugh, RN, BSN, CPN
Clinical Education Coordinator
Pediatrics

Sandra L. Lederman, RN, C, BSN
Research Nurse
Cystic Fibrosis

Lizette LeVieux-Anglin, RN, MS
Clinical Nurse Specialist
Pediatric Surgery

Jean Pool, RN, C, MSN
Educator
Pediatrics

Leslie H. Saunders. RN, C, MS
Clinical Nurse Specialist
Pediatrics

Laurie Ann K. Woo, RN, MS
Instructor of Nursing and Staff Nurse II,
Pediatric Ward, PICU

CONTRIBUTORS

Angela Atkinson, RN, MSN
Unit Educator, Hematology-Oncology
Texas Children's Hospital
Houston, Texas

Cynthia R. Baker, RN, BSN
Staff Nurse
Texas Children's Hospital
Houston, Texas

Trilla A. Batts, CCRN, ARNP, MSN
Pediatric Educator
University Medical Center
Faculty Affiliation with
University of Florida
Jacksonville, Florida

Debra L. Berdy, RN, BSN
Nursing Instructor/Staff Nurse
Children's Hospital Medical Center of Akron
Akron, Ohio

Diane Bergh, RN, MS
Instructor, Nursing
University of Hawaii
Nurse Educator/CNS
Kapiolani Medical Center for
Women & Children
Honolulu, Hawaii

Susan D. Beyer, RN, BSN
Unit Educator, Neurosurgery/Neurology
Texas Children's Hospital
Houston, Texas

Leslie A. Biddinger, RN, MS, CPN
Unit Educator
Texas Children's Hospital
Houston, Texas

Janis R. Boatright, RN, BS
Unit Educator, Pediatric ICU
Texas Children's Hospital
Houston, Texas

Valerie Y. Brannon, RN, C, BSN, MS
Nurse Manager
Texas Children's Hospital
Houston, Texas

Carol A. Brave, RN, BSN
Staff Nurse, Pediatric Critical Care
St. Louis Children's Hospital
St. Louis, Missouri

Janet M. Brucker, RN, MS, CNRN
Assistant Director, Nursing
Texas Children's Hospital
Houston, Texas

June Chan, RN, MSN
Director, Nursing Practice and Research
Children's Hospital of the King's Daughters
Norfolk, Virginia

Judith Conedera, RN, MSN
Assistant Professor, Nursing
Purdue University Calumet
Hammond, Indiana

Linda Crim, RN, BSN, CPN
Program Coordinator, HIV Program
Children's Hospital
Columbus, Ohio

Meg Danner, RN, MS
CNS, Diabetes
St. Louis Children's Hospital
St. Louis, Missouri

Nancy H. Danou, RN, MSN, CPN
Assistant Professor,
Family Health Nursing
University of Wisconsin
Eau Claire, Wisconsin

Nancy Jane Donoho, RN, C, MSN
CNS, Maternal/Infant
Fort Sanders Health System
Knoxville, Tennessee

Margaret Evelyn-Pinkser, RN, C, MA
Instructor, Staff Development & Cont. Ed.
Maimonides Medical Center
Brooklyn, New York

Denise K. Fleig, RN, MSN
CNS, Pediatric ICU
Wyler Children's Hospital at
University of Chicago Hospitals
Chicago, Illinois

Lois Jean Fredell, RN, BSN, BA
Staff Nurse
Minneapolis Children's Medical Center
Minneapolis, Minnesota

Willa Hill Fuller, RN, C, BSN
Education Coordinator
Medical/Surgical Services
Orlando Regional Healthcare System
Orlando, Florida

Jeanne Garnett, RN, CCRN
Staff Nurse
St Louis Children's Hospital
St. Louis, Missouri

Bren Groves, RN, MN
Nurse Educator
Sacred Heart General Hospital
Eugene, Oregon

Michelle R. Hicks, RN, BSN
Clinical Nurse III
C.S. Mott Children's Hospital
University of Michigan Medical Center
Ann Arbor, Michigan

Carol Frances Holt, RN, MSN, BS
CNS, Pediatric Cardiovascular
Children's Hospital
San Diego, California

Nancy G. Hoyt, RN, MN
Director of Nursing, Medical/Surgical
Salem Hospital
Salem, Oregon

Deirdre F. Jackson, RN, MSN, CRRN
CNS, Pediatric
Children's Specialized Hospital
Mountainside, New Jersey

Doris Jackson, RN, ADN
Nurse Manager
Texas Children's Hospital
Houston, Texas

Dearne L. Johnson, RN
Staff Development
Children's Hospital Medical Center of Akron
Akron, Ohio

Joanna Rowe Kaakinen, RN, PhD
Assistant Professor, Nursing
University of Portland
Portland, Oregon

Maggie Kelling, RN, BSN, M.Ed.
Senior Nursing Instructor
Children's Hospital Medical Center of Akron
Akron, Ohio

Amy Kennedy, RN, MSN
Nursing Practice Review Coordinator
St. Louis Children's Hospital
St. Louis, Missouri

Camille Kleeschulte, RN, ADN, TNCC, ABLS
Staff Nurse
St. Louis Children's Hospital
St. Louis, Missouri

Mary L. Krywanio, RN, DNS
Director, Nursing Education & Research
St. Louis Children's Hospital
St. Louis, Missouri

Denise LeBaugh, RN, BSN, CPN
Coordinator, Clinical Education
Children's Hospital
Omaha, Nebraska

Sandra L. Lederman, RN, C, BSN
Research Nurse, Cystic Fibrosis
Children's Hospital Medical Center of Akron
Akron, Ohio

Cdr. Mary M. Leemhuis, RN, BS
Assistant Chief Nurse/Nurse Educator
US Public Health Service
Carl Albert Indian Health Facility
Ada, Oklahoma

Lizette LeVieux-Anglin, RN, MS
CNS, Pediatric Surgery
Children's Hospital
Columbus, Ohio

Jeanne M. Lewis, RN, MSN, CEN
Coordinator, Critical Care Fellowship
Cooper Hospital/University Medical Center
Camden, New Jersey

Cynthia Mason, RN, BSN
Staff Nurse
Texas Children's Hospital
Houston, Texas

Corinne McCarthy, RN, MSN, CPN
Coordinator, Pediatric Outreach
Children's Hospital
San Diego, California

Pamela Ann Meinert, RN, BSN, MSN
Assistant Professor
Kent State University
East Liverpool, Ohio

Carolyn Mitchell, RN, ADN
Registered Nurse Unit Educator
Texas Children's Hospital
Houston, Texas

Carol J. Pankratz, RN, MSN
CNS, Medical-Surgical
Sacred Heart General Hospital
Eugene, Oregon

Jean Pool, RN, C, MSN
Educator
Doctors Medical Center
Modesto, California

Ann Marie Ramsey, RN, MSN, CPNP
CNS, Pediatric Otolaryngology
University of Michigan Hospitals
Ann Arbor, Michigan

Kay Ritchey, RN, MSN
Director, Nursing Education
All Children's Hospital
St. Petersburg, Florida

Donna E. Robles, RN, MS
Assistant Director, Nursing Education
Children's Hospital Medical Center of Akron
Akron, Ohio

Susan E. Ruble, RN, BSN, BS
Staff Nurse, Pediatric ICU
St. Louis Children's Hospital
St. Louis, Missouri

Leslie H. Saunders, RN, C, MS
Clinical Nurse Specialist
Children's Hospital, Inc.
Columbus, Ohio

Sonya LaVonne Scott, RN, C, MS
Educator
Texas Children's Hospital
Houston, Texas

Kathleen A. Simon, RN, DNS
Assistant Professor, Nursing
Medical University of South Carolina,
Charleston, South Carolina

Barbara D. Upton, RN, CPN
Nurse Manager, Pediatrics
San Bernardino County Medical Center
San Bernardino, California

Meredith Happ Weintraub, RN, MSN, PNP
Nurse Practitioner, Pediatric
Children's Hospital of Alabama
Birmingham, Alabama

Marilyn L. Weitzel, RN, MSN, BS
Instructor, Nursing
Akron School of Practical Nursing
Akron, Ohio

Kimberly A. Wilson, RN
Education Coordinator
Children's Hospital Medical Center of Akron
Akron, Ohio

Laurie Ann K. Woo, RN, MS
Instructor
University of San Francisco
Staff Nurse II, Pediatric Ward
Kaiser Permanente Medical Center
San Francisco, California

Elizabeth Wright, RN, C, MSN
Assistant Professor, Nursing
Kent State University
East Liverpool, Ohio

Roseann M. Zahara-Such, RN, MSN
Educational Coordinator
Children's Memorial Medical Center
Chicago, Illinois

THE McGRAW-HILL CLINICAL CARE PLAN SERIES

This book and its companions in the McGraw-Hill Clinical Care Plan series are the most current editions of the now "classic" Standard Nursing Care Plans that were first published by Mayers/El Camino in the mid-seventies. These books, in frequently updated versions, have been published continuously since that time. In those early years, as the first of their kind, they did much to stimulate nursing's early development of formalized, systematic care planning/evaluation systems in hospitals throughout most English-speaking countries. Today they continue to be a part of nursing's continuing effort to articulate and advance the knowledge base of nursing. In addition, metric conversions have been given as appropriate to facilitate global audiences.

These new editions, now published by McGraw-Hill, preserve all of the most preferred features of previous editions. They also contain many enhancements in format and style which make them even easier to use than ever before. The content has benefited from the contributions of a greater number, and wider range, of nurse caregivers, specialists, and educators than there were before.

These books maintain continuity with previous editions through oversight by the same Series Editor, Marlene Mayers. In addition, a new Associate Editor, Annette Jacobson has been added to the editorial team for this book, *Pediatric Nursing*. She is a Clinical Nurse Specialist and clinical educator for the maternal-child department of a large regional medical center.

This editorial team, in close collaboration with panels of clinical reviewers, have combined their talents to produce these definitive books of nursing care plans for the acute care setting.

The books in the McGraw-Hill Clinical Care Plan series are: *Perinatal/Neonatal Nursing, Pediatric Nursing,* and *Medical-Surgical Nursing.*

They are specifically designed to be used by nurses in the hospital setting. The three books address the acute problems that are experienced by many people at some time during their lives: before birth, through childhood, and into adulthood. These problems frequently result in hospitalization where nurses, as the predominant caregivers, provide the moment-by-moment care that assesses, nurtures, and guides them through their acute crises.

Guides for Care Planning in the Hospital Setting

These books are entitled "Clinical Care Plans" because they are carefully written in the succinct style associated with the clinical setting. They help nurses and students visualize how a functional care plan might be phrased. Some of these plans contain more items of information than a nurse might normally need for a specific patient, but they offer groups or combinations of activities from which to select the most relevant items. By referring to these already carefully crafted documents, and by adding the necessary qualifying words and phrases, a nurse can thereby efficiently produce care plans that contain both standardized and carefully individualized elements.

The plans' format is the familiar three-column design. Terminology is consistent with what is actually written in charts and on care plans in the clinical setting. Terms are succinct enough so that, with only minor modification, they can be entered into a critical pathway, a flow sheet, or into computerized information systems.

Each book includes the most commonly occurring medical diagnoses (or topics of concern) that are experienced by patients admitted to that clinical area.

Familiar Phraseology

Phraseology tends to conform to generally familiar hospital nursing form and style practices. (1) Nursing diagnoses are those developed by NANDA; (2) Outcome Criteria include action verbs that direct attention to those measurable/observable phenomena (subjective and objective) that make evaluation possible; (3) Interventions (groups/combinations of nursing activities) are phrased as directives.

Because these plans are meant to be used in the acute care setting, their terms are those of hospital nurses. Brief and succinct phrases are used rather than sentences. Outcome criteria are written in the present tense, active voice. Symbols and abbreviations common to the hospital setting are used.

Easy to Individualize

These care plans are easy to individualize because they are carefully crafted to apply to specific clinical situations. For example, the management of "Fluid Volume Deficit" (a NANDA diagnosis) for a child with leukemia will differ from fluid volume management for an adult or child with an eating disorder. Or, for example, "Altered Nutrition: Less than body requirements" is treated differently in the care plan for diabetes mellitus than it is in that for a child with biliary atresia or for an infant with cleft palate.

It is also within the individualization process that the patient's collaboration becomes vital. Involvement empowers people to become competent and knowledgeable about their health, and, thus, to become effective on their own behalf. Including the patient and family in reviewing, understanding, and amending the plan of care can make a significant difference in the outcomes of that care. It can also influence patients' long-term healthcare practices.

Excellent Reference Tools

The books are designed to be used on a daily basis. They provide easy-to-find information about clinical nursing care. When kept near at hand, for instance on the nursing unit as well as in school and hospital libraries, they serve as reminder systems — as do other reference texts and manuals. They are excellent references to use when nurses are reviewing literature as part of the periodic updates of their own standard nursing care plans.

A Clinical Care Plan prompts a nurse to address all of the relevant issues for a patient's care. It is difficult, when under the pressures of an acute care setting, to rely on human memory to recall each and every one of the variables to be addressed in a patient's situation. A responsible professional in any field uses "lists and prompts" to bolster human memory. Every caregiver, too, needs various kinds of reference and reminder systems to provide safe and effective care. Clinical Care Plans are among the best of them.

Excellent Learning Tools

The clearly organized format and graphic nonlinear design make these books excellent learning tools for hospital or school instruction. Each care plan illuminates the logic that underlies nursing practice. Nursing Diagnoses and etiologies along with their outcome criteria are specified. These, in turn, trigger groups or combinations of nursing activities that are understood to prevent, ameliorate, or resolve the underlying problems. The graphic format structures and organizes these units of information. Their relationships are made clear.

This logical framework helps students to more easily understand and to integrate the detailed information found in their major nursing texts.

Outcome Criteria for Quality Assurance/Improvement

Included are many outcome criteria that are directly linked to care assessment for quality enhancement. Clinical Care Plans typically offer several outcome criteria for each nursing diagnosis. Criteria are phrased in specific, measurable terms.

These care plans express commonly understood outcome and process criteria and thereby provide an excellent device for measuring quality and identifying accountability. With only minor modification they can be utilized as the source of outcome and process criteria for patient care evaluation tools such as those used in Total Quality Management (TQM), chart reviews, concurrent reviews, patient surveys, and so on.

Practice-Based Development

These books are the result of a process of collaboration among nurse clinicians, caregivers, and educators from across the country. Through this process, standards and practices have become integrated into a carefully organized, inductively developed, practice-based whole. Yet each book also clearly reflects the differing nursing cultures and voices that are unique to each clinical area.

Our goal has been to provide care plans that specifically address the needs of hospitalized patients. And we respectfully acknowledge the extraordinary commitment and skill of their caregivers: today's hospital nurses.

Acknowledgments

We wish to thank the following individuals for their extraordinary contributions to manuscript development: Bren Groves, Sandra Lederman, Christine Beneda, Keith Albin, Nancy Hoyt, Arlene Sperhac, Barbara Land, Penny Allmett, Cheryl Hunt, Carol Roth, and Peggy Pickens. A special note of appreciation goes to Shasta Hatter, our manuscript coordinator.

Marlene Mayers, RN, MS
Series Editor

Annette Jacobson, RN, MSN
Associate Editor

McGraw-Hill Clinical Care Plans

Pediatric Nursing

GENERAL

CONTENTS Instructions

GENERAL

INSTRUCTIONS

HOW TO USE McGRAW-HILL CLINICAL CARE PLANS

This definitive, easy-to-use reference book provides the hospital nurse or nursing student, with a fast-track approach to patient care planning. The design is easy to read, well-indexed, and gives the reader a jump start in developing an individualized plan of care.

THE FORMAT

The care plans are divided into six categories: Nursing Diagnoses, Outcome Criteria, Interventions, Rationale, Other Less Common Nursing Diagnoses, and Essential Discharge Criteria. Take each category and review the specific components contained within.

Nursing Diagnoses

NANDA nursing diagnoses are used as the standard nomenclature for these care plans. They are listed in the first, or left-hand, column of the care plan as noted below.

EDUCATION FOR DISCHARGE

...RSING DIAGNOSIS	OUTCOME CRITERIA	INTERVENTIONS
1 Knowledge Deficit (relevant healthcare needs) *r.t. lack of recall, cognitive limitation, impaired communication, depression, illiteracy, lack of exposure, withdrawal*	• Verbalizes understanding of instructions	• Describe how to use new skills, behaviors in daily living • Use open-ended questions to derive information regarding learning • Simplify information to meet the patient's/family's level of understanding or developmental age

Our example is "Knowledge Deficit" as it appears in our *Education for Discharge* care plan.

Because of shortened lengths of stay in the hospital, all relevant nursing diagnoses likely will be addressed upon admission. Otherwise, the diagnoses may be prioritized according to patient need and nurse judgment. The diagnostic *hunch* can be confirmed by reviewing those diagnoses listed under the topic, since they are most likely to characterize patient problems associated with that particular topic or medical diagnosis. Sometimes, the reader is referred to other care plans in the book that may help develop a particular plan or address a specific issue, such as *pain* or *education for discharge*.

2

The last part of the diagnostic statement is the etiology, or list of risk factors, that follows the "related to" phrase as shown. We have chosen to abbreviate the "related to" statement to *r.t.* within each care plan. A variety of potential etiology statements are listed to get you going. You will want to select the specific etiology for your patient as you begin to develop an individualized plan of care.

For example, Knowledge Deficit might be related to "lack of recall" for one patient, to "cognitive limitation" for another, to "illiteracy" for a third patient.

Clearly, the different etiologies would require different teaching-learning interventions.

EDUCATION FOR DISCHARGE

NURSING DIAGNOSIS	OUTCOME CRITERIA	INTERVENTIONS
1 **Knowledge Deficit (relevant healthcare needs)** *r.t. lack of recall, cognitive limitation, impaired communication, depression, illiteracy, lack of exposure, withdrawal*	• Verbalizes understanding of instructions	• Describe how to use new skills, behaviors in daily living • Use open-ended questions to derive information regarding learning • Simplify information to meet the patient's/family's level of understanding or developmental age

---

Outcome Criteria

The next column addresses *Outcome Criteria* which is the term chosen to reflect the goals for the patient. Here you will find the patient outcomes anticipated for the certain nursing diagnoses. The outcome, which is written in specific terms, may address the patient and/or family.

These objective and subjective criteria are written in terms of measurable patient behaviors, and each criterion identifies the patient's goals by the time of discharge. Similarly, outcome criteria include objective and subjective parameters that describe successful resolution of the nursing diagnoses.

Because the length of stay in today's acute care setting is compressed, all outcome criteria should be met during the patient's hospital stay. For clarity and simplicity, outcomes have not been separated into short- or long-term phrases. However, care plans can be used as guides for critical pathways or care maps by assigning daily goals, determined by institutional preferences and regional population needs.

You will find that the term *within normal limits* (WNL) has been used to allow for the variation of normal. That variation may be normal for that patient, i.e., return to baseline, or preadmission status. Or normal may reflect the variation within the literature. And it can reflect the variation between institutions or physician preferences for monitoring response to treatment.

EDUCATION FOR DISCHARGE

NURSING DIAGNOSIS	OUTCOME CRITERIA	INTERVENTIONS
1 Knowledge Deficit (relevant healthcare needs) *r.t. lack of recall, cognitive limitation, impaired communication, depression, illiteracy, lack of exposure, withdrawal*	• Verbalizes understanding of instructions	• Describe how to use new ▨▨▨ behaviors in daily living • Use open-ended questions ▨ derive information regarding learning • Simplify information to meet the patient's/family's level of understanding or developmental age

Interventions

Nursing actions are listed in the third column. *Interventions* identify independent and interdependent strategies designed to facilitate or accomplish the outcome criteria. Interventions are specific enough to ensure that established standards of clinical practice are met, yet general enough to allow for institutional preferences. Monitoring and assessment strategies are listed to guide the nurse in ascertaining that outcomes have been met.

Actions listed are both independent and interdependent. Suggestions for referrals are stated when the plan of care may require the expertise of another healthcare discipline. The care plan format can be easily adapted to document which interventions were provided by each discipline. For instance, the nurse can reinforce the plans set forth by the social worker, while saving time in redundant efforts.

In this column you may find the term *within parameters*. This term was chosen to address those assessments that a physician or other primary care provider may state as an acceptable range of normal, such as in blood gases or blood glucose levels. (You may want to refer to the appendixes for normative data.)

Many plans include specific teaching content to correct knowledge deficits and enhance important self-care strategies. You may want to refer to the *Education for Discharge* care plan to supplement this section.

Rationale

Listed at the end of the *Intervention* column you will find *Rationale* for the interventions as they relate to the nursing diagnosis and etiologies. These statements are simple, concise, and offer key concepts to use in researching these concepts further.

EDUCATION FOR DISCHARGE

NURSING DIAGNOSIS	OUTCOME CRITERIA	INTERVENTIONS
	• Participates in care activities	• Establish an environment that enables patient/family to gain control
		• Build on patient's developmental and learning level; consult with expert as indicated

RATIONALE: *Learning activities that are geared to the patient's/family's level of prior experience, knowledge, and developmental level are likely to produce positive cognitive behavior changes that are relevant to healthcare needs. Repetition, participation, and graphic/written cues and lists foster learning and recall.*

Other Less Common Nursing Diagnoses

Next you will find that we have included a listing of other diagnoses that tend to be associated with the medical diagnosis or problem. These diagnoses may also reflect other potential problems that patients with this medical condition present in the acute care setting.

You will see that etiologies have been omitted from the diagnostic statement, allowing for individual variations in patient assessment by the nurse. These additional nursing diagnoses, supported by a particular patient's characteristics and etiology, can be developed through the nursing process.

We refer to these diagnoses as "less common" because they are less likely to be addressed during a brief hospital stay. However, these nursing diagnoses may be commonly addressed with complications or in the outpatient or home care setting.

Essential Discharge Criteria

The final section in each care plan is the *Essential Discharge Criteria*. Here you will find that we have broadly summarized the Outcome Criteria contained within the care plan. The outcome criteria have been collapsed into essential aspects that

EDUCATION FOR DISCHARGE

OTHER LESS COMMON NURSING DIAGNOSES: *Anxiety; Ineffective Individual Coping; Noncompliance; Social Isolation; Self-Esteem Disturbance*

ESSENTIAL DISCHARGE CRITERIA

- Patient/family verbalize and/or demonstrate specific knowledge, behavior, skills relevant to condition

- Demonstrates knowledge relevant to condition: pathophysiology, prognosis, expected course of recovery

- Verbalizes, discusses specific knowledge relevant to healthcare needs: treatment plans and their rationale, potential complications and s/s to report

- Demonstrates competence in use of required equipment, assistive devices

- Verbalizes/demonstrates safe and effective use of prescribed medications

- Identifies potential drug or food interactions to be avoided

- Verbalizes realistic plans to integrate required dietary modifications into normal family diet

- Possesses follow-up appointments for required treatments and healthcare supervision

must be present to allow for a safe and effective discharge from the acute care setting.

For example, you will notice that we have assumed that basic physiologic function is present but we will speak to the need for "resolution of respiratory compromise" for the patient who was admitted with pneumonia. You won't necessarily find discussion of HR WNL, BP WNL, or bowel function WNL, since these are only indirectly related to the presenting problem. And maybe that patient has a superimposed cardiac abnormality that will not be ameliorated by the care provided during the bout with pneumonia.

Additionally, we incorporated JCAHO requirements regarding discharge. You will find strategies to ensure compliance in the *Education for Discharge* plan, which addresses Knowledge Deficit.

GETTING STARTED

Now that you have an understanding of the layout and content, it's time to get started developing your individualized care plan.

- Select the medical diagnoses you are interested in and turn to the standard care plan.

- Identify the nursing diagnosis relevant to your patient based on your assessment. Remember to review the *Other Less Common Nursing Diagnoses* section for other potential diagnoses.

- Select the appropriate etiology for each nursing diagnosis.
- Identify outcome criteria specific to the etiology demonstrated by the patient.
- Review the essential discharge criteria to ensure inclusion of essential aspects.
- List interventions necessary to facilitate achieving the identified outcomes as they relate to the patient.
- Review the plan of care with the patient and family and revise as needed.
- Implement the plan of care, communicating with other healthcare providers.
- Evaluate the patient's progress toward attaining the outcome criteria; revise the plan as needed.
- Identify variances for developing Improvement of Organizational Program (quality assurance).

HELPFUL HINTS

A successful plan begins with a solid nursing admission data base. Objective and subjective information is clustered to determine whether or not defining characteristics support a particular nursing diagnosis.

You will not find *exact* wording from care plan to care plan concerning a specific nursing diagnoses, e.g., impaired skin integrity. This is intentional, providing the reader with a variety of phrasing options. (It's also less boring that way!)

You will find the term *family* is used broadly to describe persons significant to the patient. These persons may be mother, brother, father, aunt, neighbor, friend, or any other "significant other."

For diagnoses that tend to span age groups, such as meningitis, the reader needs to incorporate developmental considerations as indicated. Additionally, the diagnosis may occur across the life span, and these developmental "passages" should be considered as well.

Achievement of Essential Discharge Criteria should be addressed and documented as part of the discharge notation. The behaviors listed are those that the patient must demonstrate before safely leaving the hospital. The nurse obtains data from ongoing patient assessment, return demonstrations, and the patient record to evaluate whether outcome criteria have been met. If the criteria are not met, appropriate referrals should be made and documented to ensure care continuity after discharge.

Appendixes may be helpful to you when looking for abbreviations, normal lab values, listing of NANDA nursing diagnoses, definitions of medical problems, or defining characteristics of NANDA diagnoses.

GENERAL

CHEMOTHERAPY

NURSING DIAGNOSES	OUTCOME CRITERIA	INTERVENTIONS
1 High Risk for Fluid Volume Deficit *r.t. vomiting and diarrhea*	• Experiences minimal nausea and vomiting	• Administer antiemetics beginning ½ h before chemotherapy administration, and continuing q4h throughout treatment • Minimize external stimuli which may exacerbate the noxious stimuli smell (no food or perfume odors) • Provide small, frequent, bland snacks
	• Experiences minimal diarrhea	• Monitor effectiveness of antidiarrheal medications • Avoid high cellulose foods and fruits • Provide small frequent feedings • Decrease or eliminate meat

	• Displays signs of balanced fluid status
	  - moist mucous membranes
	  - good skin turgor
	  - strong BP and pulse
	  - good peripheral pulses
		• Monitor I&O q4h
		• Assess VS and pulses q2-4h
		• Weigh daily
		• Monitor electrolytes daily
		• Assess skin turgor, mucous membrane integrity q2-4h
		• Report any abnormalities

		RATIONALE: *Adequate fluid balance is essential for maintaining electrolyte homeostasis.*

2 Altered Protection
 	
r.t. suppressed hematological system (neutropenia, thrombocytopenia, anemia)
	• Shows hematological values within acceptable ranges
	  - platelets > 25,000
	  - neutrophils > 500
	  - Hb > 10
		• Obtain daily lab values of bone marrow function
		• Report any abnormalities
		• Administer blood products as ordered; monitor/document effectiveness

	• Exhibits no detectable signs of bleeding	• Check all secretions (urine, sputum, stool) for occult or frank blood • Assess oral cavity q8h for s/s of bleeding • Assess extremities q8h for petechiae • Minimize/avoid all invasive procedures

NURSING DIAGNOSES	OUTCOME CRITERIA	INTERVENTIONS

	OUTCOME CRITERIA	INTERVENTIONS

	• Exhibits no s/s of infection
	  - afebrile
	  - no localized erythema, bleeding
		• Monitor temperature q4h
		
		• Assess for IV site erythema, bleeding
		
		• Institute protective isolation techniques when neutrophil count is < 500
		  - no live plant or standing water in room
		  - no invasive procedures
		  - no one with s/s of a cold or infection to enter room
		
		• Administer anti-pyretics regularly

		RATIONALE: *Chemotherapy suppresses bone marrow, increasing the risk for bleeding and infection.*
3 Altered Oral Mucous Membrane *r.t. effects of chemotherapy*	• Displays minimum mucosal membrane breakdown	• Assess oral mucosa q8h for redness, swelling, ulceration, and candidiasis • Observe for difficulty swallowing, drooling, and signs of pain • Institute q2h normal saline oral rinses; rinse after every emesis • Use soft toothbrush or toothettes for oral care
	• Swallows and talks without pain	• Explore use of oral topical anesthetics for pain • Initiate antiacid for epigastric reflux and associated pain • Encourage child to suck on ice chips • Avoid spicy, hot foods or medications in an alcohol base
	• Displays no signs of *C. albicans*	• Assess oral mucosa q8h for candidiasis (fuzzy white patches) • Administer oral antifungal medications as ordered
		RATIONALE: *Chemotherapy breaks down integrity of epithelial lining, predisposing patient to infection.*

> ### OTHER LESS COMMON NURSING DIAGNOSES:
> *Anxiety; High Risk for Injury; Altered Family Processes; Body Image Disturbance*

ESSENTIAL DISCHARGE CRITERIA

- Maintains balanced, sufficient fluid volume

- Displays no s/s of infection or bleeding

- Parent/child explain s/s of infection and bleeding

- Parent/child perform oral hygiene sufficient to maintain oral comfort

EDUCATION FOR DISCHARGE

NURSING DIAGNOSES	OUTCOME CRITERIA	INTERVENTIONS
1 Knowledge Deficit (relevant healthcare needs) *r.t. lack of recall, cognitive limitation, impaired communication, illiteracy, lack of exposure, withdrawal, depression*	• Verbalizes understanding of instructions	• Describe how to use new skills, behaviors in daily living • Use open-ended questions to derive information regarding learning • Simplify information to meet the patient's/family's level of understanding or developmental age
	• Demonstrates appropriate decision-making	• Discuss healthcare needs and methods to achieve success • Teach use of cues to remember health actions • Assess knowledge deficit at every interaction • Consult as needed to develop appropriate teaching plan for patient/family with neurologic learning deficits
	• Assumes responsibility for own learning	• Contact patient/family to provide support; evaluate learning
	• Participates in care activities	• Establish an environment that enables patient/family to gain control • Build on patient's developmental and learning level; consult with expert as indicated
	• Possesses phone numbers for emergency medical help	• Provide opportunities for patient/family to be actively involved in learning • Assess satisfaction with education plan • Provide written materials to reinforce teaching

RATIONALE: *Learning activities that are geared to the patient's/family's level of prior experience, knowledge, and developmental level are likely to produce positive cognitive behavior changes that are relevant to healthcare needs. Repetition, participation, and graphic/written cues and lists foster learning and recall.*

GENERAL

NURSING DIAGNOSES	OUTCOME CRITERIA	INTERVENTIONS
2 Knowledge Deficit (specific knowledge, skills, behaviors) *r.t. lack of future orientation, impaired communication, anger, insufficient maturation to comprehend, refusal to listen*	• Demonstrates skills, behaviors correctly	• Provide information at level of learner's understanding • Utilize self-care protocols and/or instructional packets (as available)
	• Demonstrates ability to perform care	• Set clear learning goals • Utilize motivational techniques to assist patient/family to self-identify necessity of skill
	• Asks questions; seeks clarification	• Provide opportunity to review process or concepts related to skills, behaviors • Discuss realistic expectations to assist in guiding learning
	• Makes realistic statements about expected course, recovery, prognosis	• Offer peer support network or opportunity to observe others successfully mastering care skills and symptom control • Facilitate sense of mastery of skills, behaviors, attitudes
		RATIONALE: *Mutual goal-setting, positive feedback, and return demonstrations motivate the learner to gain desired competencies. The support of significant others also fosters motivation.*

3 Knowledge Deficit (medications)
 	
r.t. lack of exposure, irrational beliefs, need to make sense of life-threatening disease, inability to recall
	• Acquires knowledge of medication administration
	  - lists medications
	  - discusses dosages, effects, side effects
		• Provide opportunity to gain sense of control
		  - provide instruction in several modalities
		• Anticipate and provide assists when sensory or psychomotor limitations are present

	• Verbalizes knowledge of complications	• Provide written and/or audiovisual materials to enable review by patient/family as needed
	• Lists reportable s/s	• Assess patient's/family's acceptance of diagnosis • If available, help patient/family to learn computerized monitoring systems, e.g., OneTouch, Accucheck

NURSING DIAGNOSES	OUTCOME CRITERIA	INTERVENTIONS
		• Discuss sign of decrease in symptoms and/or improvement in health state
	• Discusses rationale for treatment	• Use patient's/family's ideas about illness as a starting point for education and/or training
		RATIONALE: *Use of various teaching-learning modalities that stimulate cognitive, affective, and motor abilities reinforces new and accurate information. Clear, specific information, accompanied by cues and lists, fosters recall of important information.*

GENERAL

4 Knowledge Deficit (diet) *r.t. lack of interest in learning, lack of belief in efficacy of treatment, decreased motivation to learn, misinterpretation of information*	• Demonstrates prescribed diet planning - selects indicated foods from list - recognizes contraindicated foods	• Describe problem-solving process to assist patient/family to integrate diet plan • Discuss with other healthcare providers the need to actively involve patient/family in decision-making • Establish an environment conducive to learning - free of distraction - with visual aids and diet lists • Teach how to provide rewards for maintenance of positive health behaviors
	• Verbalizes knowledge of follow-up appointments	• Reinforce utilization of information gained - include support persons in integration of information • Teach patient/family how to find, use, and evaluate community resources - education - support - treatment

NURSING DIAGNOSES	OUTCOME CRITERIA	INTERVENTIONS
	• Copes adequately	• Discuss plans for patient/family to include health behaviors identified as valuable to self
		• Set clear, mutually agreed-upon learning goals
		• Be accessible to patient/family to reinforce teaching
		RATIONALE: *Involvement in anticipatory problem-solving and planning raises likelihood of effective problem-solving after discharge. Discussion by patient and family of coping strengths and healthcare goals raises the likelihood of a continuation of this kind of support network. Discussion and support foster effective behavior changes.*
5 Knowledge Deficit (equipment) *r.t. excessive anxiety, need to follow new and/or complex treatment, unfamiliarity with information*	• Demonstrates competence in equipment use	• Teach how to mentally and physically rehearse skill
		• Describe how mastery meets patient's/family's own standard for adequate coping
	• Possesses phone numbers for equipment and supplies	• Demonstrate to patient/family how to use equipment and obtain services
		• Discuss where to access supplies and/or equipment; provide written information
	• Demonstrates required skills related to supplies required	• Assist with practice of skill until performance shows mastery and confidence
	• Verbalizes understanding of instructions	• Check with patient/family often during teaching to elicit and evaluate understanding
		RATIONALE: *Demonstration and return demonstration with positive, supportive feedback enhance motor skill mastery.*

> ***OTHER LESS COMMON NURSING DIAGNOSES:*** *Anxiety; Ineffective Individual Coping; Noncompliance; Social Isolation; Self-Esteem Disturbance*

ESSENTIAL DISCHARGE CRITERIA

- Patient/family verbalize and/or demonstrate specific knowledge, behavior, skills relevant to condition

- Demonstrates knowledge relevant to condition: pathophysiology, prognosis, expected course of recovery

- Verbalizes, discusses specific knowledge relevant to healthcare needs: treatment plans and their rationale; potential complications and s/s to report

- Demonstrates competence in use of required equipment, assistive devices

- Verbalizes/demonstrates safe and effective use of prescribed medications

- Identifies potential drug or food interactions to be avoided

- Verbalizes realistic plans to integrate required dietary modifications into normal family diet

- Possesses follow-up appointments for required treatments and healthcare supervision

GENERAL

GRIEF

NURSING DIAGNOSES	OUTCOME CRITERIA	INTERVENTIONS
1 Anticipatory Grieving *r.t. impending or actual loss of child or the loss of child's functions or capacities*	• Child/family express feelings as freely as they desire	• Assess for s/s of normal grieving - denial of loss - emotional numbness - anxiety - somatic s/s such as hyperventilation, sighing, restlessness, or weakness - transient confusion, disorientation - crying - anger • Provide time and private space for active listening - encourage expression of feelings - avoid "smoothing over" or distraction from loss
	• Child/family explain, express the meaning of the loss within their context	• Assist child/family to identify the loss and discuss its meaning within the context of their lives, hopes, other problems • Explain the need for time to pass in order to adapt to the loss
	• Child/family experience early identification, appropriate support for unhealthy coping behaviors - substance abuse - persistent expression of guilt and/or self-recrimination - aggression toward self or others	• Assess for signs of unhealthy coping behaviors • Report and intervene, if needed, to prevent injury • Make referral to appropriate counseling resource • Recognize cultural differences
		RATIONALE: *Displaying acceptance of grief is an essential first step in helping the family cope with the loss. Encouraging the parents' verbalization of the specific meanings of the loss within helps them to identify the other stressors in their life situation. This understanding helps them to identify their strengths and unique coping abilities.*
2 Fear *r.t. emotional upheaval and "unknowns" of dying process*	• Child/family identify specific fears	• Assess the individual family members' grieving and their coping styles • Provide "permission" to express their fears by expressing what others in similar situations have shared with you

NURSING DIAGNOSES	OUTCOME CRITERIA	INTERVENTIONS
		• Give positive feedback regarding their strengths and coping mechanisms
		• Avoid forcing child/family members to confront emotional issues; respect their stage of the grief process
		• Help child/family members identify specific fears and talk about them
	• Child/family use appropriate support systems and resources	• Identify the family's support systems and assist in planning for mobilizing those resources
		• Stay with and provide companionship as possible
		• Provide brief, clear explanations when there is unexpected worsening of child's situation; do so even if parents are unresponsive
		• Facilitate inclusion of family's support persons or spiritual advisor
		• Allow family and significant others to see the child before and after death
		RATIONALE: *Mobilizing the parents' support systems reduces their isolation. Companionship, or quietly being with the parents, reduces isolation and fear. The child, even though gravely ill, is aware that his parents are with him and comforting him. This caring communication reduces fear of the situation.*
3 Altered Family Processes *r.t. imminent death of child*	• Parents/family members participate in care as condition permits	• Encourage family members to participate in care • Liberalize visiting policies • Allow for personal, private time for the child and family
	• Parents/family share their feelings and concerns with each other	• Foster family dialogue - offer to initiate issues for discussion - promote face-to-face communication among the family members

NURSING DIAGNOSES	OUTCOME CRITERIA	INTERVENTIONS
	• Parents/family members appear physically rested most of the time	• Explain the need for caring for their own health; the need for rest, exercise, good nutrition • Suggest rotating bedside time among the family members so there can be periods of emotional and physical relief for each family member

RATIONALE: *Open discussion of sensitive issues is fostered by a catalyst (a nurse or counselor) who is not burdened by a family's past, long-standing role expectations, guilt, and misunderstandings. Periodic breaks and rest periods are important, reducing the physical and emotional exhaustion from constant attendance at the bedside.*

OTHER LESS COMMON NURSING DIAGNOSES: *High Risk for Caregiver Role Strain; Powerlessness; Spiritual Distress; Family Coping: Potential for growth*

ESSENTIAL DISCHARGE CRITERIA

• Child/family share feelings with one another

• Parents have secured help for any unhealthy coping behaviors

• Family displays reliance on needed support persons or systems

• Parents have participated in child's care to the extent possible

• Parents express caring communication and touching with the child before and after death as culturally appropriate

PAIN MANAGEMENT

NURSING DIAGNOSES	OUTCOME CRITERIA	INTERVENTIONS

1 Pain
r.t. surgery and/or disease process
	• Demonstrates reduced or minimal pain
	  - able to participate in ADL
	  - rests comfortably
	  - verbalizes decreased pain intensity
	  - maintains heart rate and BP WNL
		• Evaluate child's autonomic responses for increased heart rate and increased BP
		
		• Observe for moaning, crying, grimacing, restlessness, and guarding
		
		• If developmentally appropriate, encourage the child to describe pain using a scale such as the Wong & Baker scale, or to rate pain intensity on scale from 1-10
		
		• Provide diversional activities, such as television, books, games, and bubbles; assist with imagery techniques that help alleviate pain intensity
		
		• Administer pain medications by mouth or into an IV line whenever possible; evaluate effectiveness
		
		RATIONALE: *Consistent pain management produces sustained comfort, allowing the child to rest more comfortably.*

2 Anxiety
r.t. misconceptions about pain
	• Verbalizes or demonstrates decreased anxiety
	  - participates in care
	  - cries less
	  - plays more
	  - interacts with staff
	  - expresses concerns about pain
		• If developmentally appropriate, upon admission explain essentials of pain management (types of pain medications, when to request medications, alternative methods for alleviating pain)
		
		• When obtaining admission history, inquire about past experiences with pain
		
		• Allow time for child to ask questions, express concerns about pain
		
		• Explain to child and parents the procedures or treatments that elicit pain
		
		• If appropriate, incorporate play when explaining painful procedures or treatments
		
		• Have someone stay with child during painful procedures or treatments per institutional standards

NURSING DIAGNOSES	OUTCOME CRITERIA	INTERVENTIONS
		• If possible, always anticipate the patient's need for pain medication (before or after therapy, during a dressing change, or prior to painful procedures) • Avoid fearful statements, such as, "I am going to give you a shot for pain" • Give child control whenever possible (taking off bandages, choosing injection site, holding equipment)
		RATIONALE: *Verbalizing perceptions of past and current pain reduces the child's anxiety. Learning from past experiences with pain helps the child to successfully manage current pain. Explanations and the presence of supportive persons reduce fear, thus minimizing perceptions of pain.*
3 Knowledge Deficit *r.t. pain management*	• Parent/child verbalize and demonstrate an understanding of pain and its management - participation in care - proper demonstration of diversional activities - appropriate selection of analgesics for controlling various types of pain	• Assess parent's/child's understanding of pain management • Allow parent/child time to verbalize questions, concerns about pain management • Devise an individualized teaching plan that is developmentally appropriate; instructions include - causes of pain - description of pain - how to effectively manage pain - medications and methods of administration - a list of diversional activities • Provide time for the child to practice diversional techniques - deep breathing - splinting - positioning
		RATIONALE: *Individualized and consistent pain management that incorporates pharmacological and nonpharmacological techniques provides sustained comfort.*

OTHER LESS COMMON NURSING DIAGNOSES:
Activity Intolerance; Constipation; Self-Esteem Disturbance

ESSENTIAL DISCHARGE CRITERIA

- Displays evidence of sustained or reasonable comfort

- Parent/child demonstrate ability to manage an established pain control regimen

RADIATION THERAPY

NURSING DIAGNOSES	OUTCOME CRITERIA	INTERVENTIONS
1 High Risk for Impaired Skin Integrity *r.t. radiation-induced changes*	• Maintains intact skin tissues; skin markings intact	• Inspect skin daily for breakdown • Keep treated area clean and dry • Wash the treated area with warm water and mild soap or shampoo daily; rinse soap off thoroughly • Dry the treated area using gentle patting motions with a soft clean towel • Keep skin folds dry; expose these areas to air when possible • Do not apply cosmetics, creams, deodorant, lotions, ointments, perfume, powders, tape, or any substance in the treated area • Avoid exposure of treated area to heating pads, hot water bottles, high-heat hair dryers, sunlamps, direct sunlight, ice packs, and extremes in environmental temperature • Protect the treated area from friction, rubbing, and itching; avoid massaging treated area • Wear loose-fitting cotton clothing over treated skin normally covered by clothing
	• Parent/child perform skin care and state s/s of side effects	• Instruct about skin markings, potential side effects, general skin care
		RATIONALE: *Appropriate care can help minimize trauma and irritation of the treated skin.*

2 Knowledge Deficit
 	
r.t. radiation therapy and management of child's care
	• Parent/child discuss radiation therapy
	  - goal of radiation therapy
	  - expected course of treatment
	  - radiation treatment procedure
	  - side effects of treatment and what and when to report to medical staff
		• Explain the goal of radiation therapy, the procedure, possible side effects, and complications to report

NURSING DIAGNOSES	OUTCOME CRITERIA	INTERVENTIONS

		• Describe procedure of radiation treatments
		  - simulation
		  - skin markings/tatoos
		  - plaster casts/molds
		  - treatment procedure
		
		• Review treatment schedule
		
		• Describe the expected and potential side effects of radiation therapy specific to the area being treated
		
		• Instruct child/caregiver in action to be taken if evidence of any side effect is noted
		
		• Allow sufficient time during each teaching session for questions; clarify misconceptions
		
		• Provide specific printed material of radiation therapy, treatment schedule, and side effects

RATIONALE: *Teaching/learning increases compliance and decreases complications and costs.*

3 Anxiety

r.t. concerns about radiation therapy treatments

	• Parent/child express concerns, ask questions, report increasing comfort with radiation therapy treatment plan and care	• Ask child/parent about their questions and any concerns regarding radiation therapy • Answer questions and clarify misconceptions • Orient child/parent to radiation therapy room, equipment, and staff
	• Parent/child verbalize accurate information, realistic expectations of radiation therapy	• Instruct parent/child about radiation therapy • Refer to support groups and others who have received radiation and have adjusted well to treatment

RATIONALE: *Knowledge of what to expect and verbalization of feelings can lessen the intensity and duration of fear and anxiety.*

GENERAL

NURSING DIAGNOSES	OUTCOME CRITERIA	INTERVENTIONS
4 Altered Oral Mucous Membranes *r.t. radiation to head and neck*	• Maintains a comfortable, functional oral cavity - pink, moist, and intact mucosa, tongue, and lips - absence of inflammation and lesions - absence of infection - comfort in swallowing and talking	• Provide care regimen qid to prevent infection • Perform mouth care q2h and twice at night for severe stomatitis • Use soft toothbrush or disposable foam swabs • Perform frequent rinsing with mouthwash preparations of salt and baking soda or warm saline • Use no commercial mouthwashes or products containing alcohol or phenol • Encourage frequent fluid intake; avoid extremes in beverage and food temperature
		RATIONALE: *Prophylactic mouth care will help minimize side effects of trauma to oral mucosa, tongue, and lips.*
5 Altered Nutrition: Less than body requirements *r.t. radiation therapy to abdomen, pelvis, or lower back inducing nausea and vomiting and/or malabsorption of GI tract*	• Maintains body weight at least 90% of normal for height, frame	• Monitor weight daily
	• Consumes a well-balanced, high-protein, high-calorie diet	• Instruct and assist parent/child in selection of high-protein, high-calorie foods • Instruct caregiver to avoid overemphasis on eating • Monitor and document oral intake • Instruct parent/child of the importance of oral hygiene before meals to enhance taste
	• Has no nausea or vomiting	• Offer frequent, small meals and snacks • Administer antiemetics before radiation therapy treatment and as ordered
		RATIONALE: *Several small meals and snacks are less fatiguing and tolerated better than large meals. Prevention of nausea and vomiting enhances appetite.*

NURSING DIAGNOSES	OUTCOME CRITERIA	INTERVENTIONS
Diarrhea *r.t. radiation therapy to pelvis, lower back, abdomen inducing bowel mucosa irritation*	• Maintains a normal pattern of bowel movements - stools are formed - no abdominal pain - no more than three stools per day - serum electrolytes are within normal limits	• Monitor stools, document - frequency - amount - consistency - color • Monitor I&O • Monitor electrolytes • Obtain stool for cultures and studies as ordered • Administer antidiarrheal agents as ordered • Provide bland, low-residue, lactose-free diet • Provide optimal fluid intake
	• Is free of anal excoriation	• Inspect anal mucosa daily • Provide daily sitz baths • Prohibit rectal temperatures or suppositories

RATIONALE: *Prevention, early detection, and prompt treatment decrease side effects from irritation of bowel mucosa.*

> **OTHER LESS COMMON NURSING DIAGNOSES:** *Pain; High Risk for Infection; Fatigue; Body Image Disturbance; Impaired Swallowing; Altered Sexuality Patterns; Altered Urinary Elimination; High Risk for Fluid Volume Deficit*

ESSENTIAL DISCHARGE CRITERIA

- Displays intact skin; if skin breakdown, it is healing
- Tolerates diet
- Parent/child select appropriate foods that child can tolerate, retain
- Is free of or controls diarrhea and vomiting

- Parent/child discuss radiation therapy
  - goal
  - treatment schedule
  - side effects and precautions
  - who and when to call regarding complications
- Parent/child demonstrate skin and mouth care regimen

GENERAL

PREOPERATIVE CARE

1 Anxiety

r.t. separation from parents or peers; lack of understanding of purpose or outcome of procedure; anxiety about hospital environment; fear of pain, loss of mobility, mutilation, death, or other surgical risks

Outcome Criteria:

- Exhibits reduced anxiety before surgery
  - relaxed facial expressions
  - open body language
  - makes eye contact, acts trusting of staff

Interventions:

- Assess the child's previous experience and current level of understanding before beginning training
- Encourage parents to stay with child as much as possible; if hospital procedures permit, allow visits by "best friends," siblings
- Allow parents to remain with child until anesthesia has occurred
- Use language and concepts appropriate to the child's development and hospital experience
- Introduce anxiety-laden information (for example, injections) near the end of a discussion
- Reassure the child his/her privacy will be respected

Outcome Criteria:

- Parents identify location of recovery area, describe a specific plan for visiting
- Parent/child verbalize knowledge of and can cooperate with pre- and post-op procedures

Interventions:

- Orient parents/child to the hospital environment, routines, and any special procedures planned for the child

---

Outcome Criteria:

- Listens, asks age-appropriate questions

- Verbalizes age-appropriate understanding of anticipated events

Interventions:

- Use visual aids to describe the procedure; a simple line drawing of a boy or girl is often helpful
  - emphasize that no other body part will be involved in surgery
  - emphasize the temporary nature of casts, bandages, scars, etc.
  - if a body part is associated with a specific function, stress that normal functions will not change (for example, after a tonsillectomy, child can still speak)
  - emphasize rewards at end of procedure, such as going home, seeing parent

NURSING DIAGNOSES	OUTCOME CRITERIA	INTERVENTIONS

	• Experiments with environment and required procedures	• Allow child to have the maximum control permitted by circumstances
		  - make sure he/she knows how to make menu choices, close bed curtains, etc.
		  - allow child to decide whether parents should be present during treatment or testing procedures
		• Explain pre- and post-op routines
		• Encourage child to practice those procedures which will require cooperation, such as coughing, deep breathing, incentive spirometry

	• Displays decreased tension
	  - relaxed body posture
	  - smiles, interacts
	  - asks questions
		• Encourage expression of feelings
		  - observe child's body language, facial expressions for signs of stress or fear
		  - ask child if he/she is worried
		  - acknowledge fears and risks
		• Discuss anticipated events
		  - anesthesia
		  - postoperative experience
		  - clarify misunderstandings
		  - answer questions
		• Accept regressive behaviors; let parents know that such behaviors are normal and will eventually pass
		• Allow child to have toys, photos, good luck charms, or other comfort objects

		RATIONALE: *Psychological preparation of the child and parents reduces fear and anxiety, thus reducing the risk of postoperative complications.*

2 Altered Health Maintenance
 	
r.t. changes in usual nutritional, elimination, and comfort patterns
	• Experiences minimal disruption of normal biological patterns
	  - exhibits normal fluid and electrolyte balance
	  - resumes oral intake as soon as possible
		• Inform parents/child of the amount of time the child will be NPO
		  - explain in advance when preoperative fast will begin; let him/her have a snack before time begins
		  - explain dangers of noncompliance (if such explanation is appropriate to the child's level of readiness)
		  - let parents know when child can have food again

GENERAL

NURSING DIAGNOSES	OUTCOME CRITERIA	INTERVENTIONS
	• Sleeps, rests at normal intervals • Is awake, alert, interactive at normal times	• Plan nursing procedure and treatment at intervals that allow extended periods of rest or sleep
	• Exhibits normal VS, body temperature	• Reduce the possibility of nosocomial infection - use universal precautions - use caution in staff assignments • Instruct child about sanitary measures he/she must follow; be tactful but specific • Perform preoperative bath as per institutional standards • Perform procedures, treatments as close as possible to anticipated time; allow sufficient time for questions, interruptions, and unscheduled events
	• Displays, verbalizes sense of comfort - no guarding - relaxed body posture, facial expression	• Whenever possible, initiate intrusive or painful procedures (IV lines, NG tubes, Foley catheter) after initial anesthesia has been administered • Teach child to report unusual pains or other important s/s - use specific language appropriate to the child's development - discuss importance of pain as a diagnostic tool - emphasize that reporting important symptoms is not whining or "wimping out" - during preoperative preparations, encourage child to report pain by asking if painful procedures hurt; ignore stoic responses

RATIONALE: *Optimal physiological balance decreases incidence of postoperative complications. Careful hygiene and aseptic techniques prevent postoperative infections by reducing chance of microbial invasion, transmission, or proliferation.*

NURSING DIAGNOSES	OUTCOME CRITERIA	INTERVENTIONS
3 Knowledge Deficit *r.t. anxiety about surgical procedure, treatment rationale, follow-up care, and/or expected results*	• Parent/child verbalize correct understanding of surgery - discuss surgical anatomy - ask questions, express concerns	• Explain surgical anatomy; elicit questions, concerns; clarify misconceptions • Describe specific medical, nursing activities in first hours post-op and rationales for activities - use charts, diagrams, drawings, or mannequins to describe surgery - describe general postoperative course - explain expected time of ambulation, eating, playing - explain how much parents can be with child - remind that more teaching will occur after surgery
	• Parent/child display behaviors consistent with reduced anxiety - parents smile, interact, touch, hug child - family displays calm, non-agitated demeanor - family expresses appropriate optimism about expected results of surgery	• Monitor family behaviors for evidence of reduced anxiety • Provide support and opportunity to discuss cause of aniety
	• Family discusses expected home care requirements, asks questions, identifies support networks and/or persons	• Review home care: special procedures, diet, pain, activity, follow-up; make referrals as needed; refer to support persons as indicated

RATIONALE: *Knowledge provides the ability to predict future events, which reduces anxiety and promotes learning.*

GENERAL

OTHER LESS COMMON NURSING DIAGNOSES: *Pain; Fear; Family Coping: Potential for growth*

ESSENTIAL DISCHARGE CRITERIA

• Not applicable

POSTOPERATIVE CARE

NURSING DIAGNOSES	OUTCOME CRITERIA	INTERVENTIONS
1 Ineffective Breathing Pattern *r.t. depressant effects of anesthesia, medications; pain; anxiety; positioning*	• Maintains normal breathing pattern and breath sounds - normal RR - clear breath sounds - normal ABGs	• Monitor and report s/s of ineffective airway clearance of breathing q15min-q2h
	• Cooperates with coughing, spirometry, positioning, activity	• Assist with coughing and deep breathing and incentive spirometry as per institutional standards • Change position q2h • Increase child's activity as allowed, tolerated • Suction secretions prn
	• Displays relaxed body posture, facial expressions	• Implement actions to decrease fear and anxiety; use comfort measures - stroking - distractions - sedatives, analgesics as indicated
		RATIONALE: *Stimulation, activity, and reduced tension help prevent respiratory complications.*
2 High Risk for Injury (internal) *r.t. postoperative bleeding*	• Shows VS, BP stable, WNL	• Monitor VS, BP q15-30min until stable then qh for 4-6h; then q4h prn
	• Maintains balanced I&O	• Maintain strict I&O
	• Shows normal Hb, Hct	• Monitor lab values
	• Shows no bright bleeding from operative site, tubes, or catheters	• Inspect operative site, dressing for bright bleeding q1-2h; reinforce if saturated; report • Inspect all drainage for evidence of bright bleeding; report
	• Exhibits no cyanosis, pallor, diaphoresis, restlessness	• Observe for shock - assess for pallor, cyanosis, restlessness, diaphoresis (per VS checking schedule) - if evidence of shock: place in Trendelenburg position; start O_2; keep IV lines open; call physician
		RATIONALE: *Frequent monitoring for bleeding, s/s of shock prompts timely management of negative trends.*

NURSING DIAGNOSES	OUTCOME CRITERIA	INTERVENTIONS

3 Pain
 	
r.t. surgery
 	
(Refer to "Pain Management" care plan)
	• Exhibits reduced or tolerable pain level
	  - VS, BP WNL
	  - no prolonged crying, moaning, distracted behavior; no guarding
	  - relaxed body posture, facial expression
	  - sleeps, naps qs for age
	  - moves, ambulates without resistance
	  - takes feedings
	  - no flushing, pallor, diaphoresis
		• Anticipate pain associated with the surgical procedure (especially in a nonverbal child)
		
		• Schedule pain meds instead of waiting to give as needed
		
		• Observe child for s/s of discomfort, such as crying, irritability, restlessness, poor response to feeding, body rigidity, facial tenseness, elevated vital signs, flushing or pallor, and diaphoresis
		
		• Administer analgesics by mouth or IV whenever possible (avoid IM)
		
		• Use supportive statements to reinforce effect of analgesic (tell child he/she will feel better in *x* amount of time)
		
		• Minimize activities that aggravate pain
		
		• Gently turn, reposition q2h and as needed
		
		• Assist with supporting the child's chest or abdominal incision by splinting with a pillow when coughing and deep breathing
		
		• Maintain calm environment

	• Learns and implements effective coping strategies according to developmental age	• Hold, rock, talk, sing to child • Provide diversion, distraction, back rubs, visual imaging, toys, music • Encourage a verbal child to express feelings
	• Parents are effective in assisting child to cope during the immediate post-op period	• Include parents in devising and providing comfort measures
		RATIONALE: *A combination of pharmacologic and non-pharmacologic measures sustains comfort and reduces pain and anxiety.*

GENERAL

NURSING DIAGNOSES	OUTCOME CRITERIA	INTERVENTIONS
4 **High Risk for Infection** *r.t. inadequate primary defenses (i.e., broken skin, traumatized tissues)*	• Shows clean, clear wound - no redness, swelling - no drainage, bleeding - no separation of edges	• Use universal precautions and proper hand-washing techniques before and after each contact with wound • Use careful wound care - keep wound clean and dry - change dressing as ordered and prn - cleanse with prescribed preparation if ordered - apply antibacterial solutions/ointments as ordered - report/document any unusual smell/appearance or drainage - pin diapers below abdominal dressing to prevent contamination as indicated • Report any redness/swelling at wound site
		RATIONALE: *Employing infection control precautions decreases the incidence of infection.*
5 **Constipation** *r.t. anesthesia, immobility*	• Passes moderate amount of soft, formed stool by post-op Day 3, then q1-2d	• Dangle, ambulate per orders • Advance diet as tolerated, encourage roughage as indicated
	• Has no nausea, vomiting, abdominal distension	• Inspect for distension q4-8h
	• Has audible bowel sounds	• Assess bowel sounds q8h; report decreased bowel sounds, distension, inadequate stooling
		RATIONALE: *Monitoring for return of bowel activity provides for early detection, management. Progressive movement, activity, and mobility hastens recovery from depressant effects of anesthesia on bowel.*

> **OTHER LESS COMMON NURSING DIAGNOSES:**
> *Altered Urinary Elimination; Fluid Volume Deficit; Impaired Skin Integrity; Fluid Volume Excess*

ESSENTIAL DISCHARGE CRITERIA

- Exhibits normal breathing pattern and clear breath sounds
- Maintains balanced I&O
- Reports, displays reasonable comfort with oral analgesia
- Has audible bowel sounds

- Displays clear, clean wound, edges approximated and closing
- Parents demonstrate competence in required postoperative care for child, verbalize s/s reportable to PCP

PREOPERATIVE CARE, INFANT

NURSING DIAGNOSES	OUTCOME CRITERIA	INTERVENTIONS
1 Anxiety (parents) *r.t. fear of surgical risks, anesthesia, outcomes*	• Parents verbalize acceptance of anesthesia, surgery	• Provide information about anesthesia, surgery - describe type of anesthesia, recovery from anesthesia - describe surgery: time to perform, time to recover, when able to see infant post-op
	• Parents verbalize fears, ask questions, make specific plans for time of first post-op visit with infant	• Provide listening, support - encourage to state perceptions - identify, clarify misconceptions - explain that worry is normal - include support persons - verify that parents know of lounges, dining areas, chapel, phones, etc. - let parents know when they can visit before and after surgery
		RATIONALE: *Surgery poses increased anxiety for many persons. These measures will help parents deal with the multiple stressors of having a child undergo surgery.*
2 Knowledge Deficit (parents) *r.t. surgery, treatment rationale, follow-up care, expected results*	• Parents discuss surgical anatomy, ask questions, express concerns	• Explain surgical anatomy; elicit questions, concerns; clarify misconceptions • Use visual material as available
	• Parents discuss early postoperative course, express appropriate optimism about expected outcomes	• Describe specific medical, nursing activities in first hours post-op: explain rationales for activities
	• Parents hold, cuddle, soothe infant	• Explain how much parents can visit; encourage holding, touching, soothing behaviors as possible
	• Parents utilize support persons who are available	• Make referrals to support persons as indicated
		RATIONALE: *This may be the first surgical experience in these parents' lives. Parents may have had information overload, making it difficult to integrate knowledge during the stress of hospitalization.*

NURSING DIAGNOSES	OUTCOME CRITERIA	INTERVENTIONS

3 Fluid Volume Deficit
 	
r.t. NPO, operative condition
	• Is well-hydrated
	  - normal BP
	  - HR WNL
	  - balanced I&O
	  - stable body weight
	  - urine output at least 1-2 mL/kg/h
	  - no vomiting, diarrhea
	  - no evaporative water loss
		• Monitor, maintain I&O
		  - assess HR, BP
		  - compare I&O qh
		  - weigh daily
		  - measure urinary output (mL/kg/h); weigh diapers; obtain sp. gr.
		  - observe for and record any vomiting, diarrhea
		  - administer ordered parenteral fluids; maintain patent IV
		  - use fluid loss barrier if in radiant warmer

	• Maintains axillary temperature 36.4-37.2°C (97.5-99°F)	• Monitor axillary temperature q2-4h or prn; provide thermal support as indicated
	• Has moist mucous membranes, good skin turgor, normal fontanel tension	• Inspect mucous membranes, skin, anterior fontanel q2h
		RATIONALE: *These assessment measures minimize potential for occurrece of radiogenic problems associated with dependence on parenteral fluid administration.*

4 High Risk for Infection
 	
r.t. preoperative preparation, preoperative clinical problem
	• Exhibits no evidence of infection
	  - has normal skin color
	  - maintains axillary temperature WNL
	  - is alert and active
	  - exhibits no apnea, bradycardia
		• Monitor, manage infection prevention
		  - assess color, noting any pallor or mottling
		  - monitor axillary temperature q2-4h; note fluctuations
		  - assess activity level; note lethargy
		  - adhere to strict handwashing
		  - use sterile technique for dressings, irrigations
		  - prohibit contact with persons with URI or other infections

		RATIONALE: *Neonates are at increased risk for infection because of their immature immune response.*

GENERAL

NURSING DIAGNOSES	OUTCOME CRITERIA	INTERVENTIONS
5 Altered Nutrition: Less than body requirements *r.t. NPO status, increased nutritional requirements*	• Shows glucose WNL	• Monitor, manage blood glucose - monitor blood glucose levels; report deviations - administer parenteral replacements, TPN per orders - maintain patent IV as ordered
	• Shows K, Ca, and Na WNL	• Monitor, manage serum Na and K - monitor levels; report deviations - administer parenteral replacements, TPN per orders - maintain patent IV

RATIONALE: *NPO status limits strategies for meeting nutritional requirements.*

> **OTHER LESS COMMON NURSING DIAGNOSES:** *Inability to Sustain Spontaneous Ventilation; Impaired Tissue Integrity; Impaired Skin Integrity; High Risk for Impaired Skin Integrity; Sleep Pattern Disturbance; Interrupted Breastfeeding; Activity Intolerance*

ESSENTIAL DISCHARGE CRITERIA

• Not applicable

NURSING DIAGNOSES	OUTCOME CRITERIA	INTERVENTIONS
1 Ineffective Breathing Pattern *r.t. perioperative anesthesia*	• Shows stable, normal VS, BP	• Monitor VS, BP q15-30min until stable, qh as indicated
	• Maintains patent airway	• Maintain airway - keep ETT, resuscitation equipment at bedside - suction prn - have mechanical ventilation available
	• Is free of s/s of pulmonary compromise - RR 40 to 60 breaths/minute - no apneic episodes - no chest retractions - breath sounds clear and equal bilaterally - pink color - pulse oximeter reading WNL - normal blood gases - clear chest x-ray	• Assess for pulmonary compromise q15min until stable, then qh - administer O_2 as needed per pulse oximeter parameters - x-ray as ordered - turn q2h as tolerated - maintain OG tube to relieve distention and promote adequate air exchange (unless contraindicated) • Assess lab values; compare with baseline - blood gases - blood glucose • Assess for central, peripheral pallor, cyanosis q15-30min until stable, then qh - minimize handling - maintain thermo-neutral environment
		RATIONALE: *Respiratory compromise is a common problem post-anesthesia, especially in the neonatal population.*
2 High Risk for Fluid Volume Deficit/Excess *r.t. perioperative fluid loss/load*	• Is free of s/s of cardiovascular compromise - regular pulse, 110-160 bpm - urinary output 1-3 mL/kg/h - normal BP - capillary refill < 3 sec - no edema	• Assess cardiovascular status q15-30min until stable, then qh; report deviations from normal limits - monitor apical pulse for irregularities, strength - monitor urinary output - monitor BP - assess capillary refill time qh - assess skin turgor, presence of edema

GENERAL

NURSING DIAGNOSES	OUTCOME CRITERIA	INTERVENTIONS
	• Experiences prompt detection of complications - normal Hb, Hct - normal serum Ca, K - normal BUN, creatinine	• Identify complications - monitor Hb, Hct lab results - monitor serum Ca, K for arrhythmia-producing deficits - monitor BUN, creatinine to assess renal function
	• Shows normal circulating volume - balanced I&O - urinary output of 1-3 mL/kg/h; urine sp. gr. of 1.003-1.015 - no vomiting; no bright bleeding from operative site	• Monitor, maintain sufficient circulating fluid volume - maintain strict I&O; administer ordered fluid replacements, volume expanders, electrolyte replacements - measure all secretions, excretions, all forms of intake/output - monitor urinary output; test sp. gr. q1-2h or as indicated - assess for vomiting and for bright bleeding related to surgical area - assess IV site for redness, edema, infiltration; ensure IV access - monitor BP q1-2h
		RATIONALE: *Fluid shifts may occur during surgery, necessitating close observation during the immediate postoperative period.*
3 Altered Nutrition: Less than body requirements *r.t. hypoglycemia, intolerance to fluid intake, hypocalcemia*	• Shows no weight loss	• Weigh daily, same scale • Assess for water retention
	• Is free of s/s of hypoglycemia, hypocalcemia - normal blood glucose and ionized Ca - no prolonged lethargy, flaccidity - no prolonged, intense irritability, tremors - alert	• Maintain IV/access, administer ordered fluids • Monitor, manage Ca, glucose levels - report deviations - assess activity level for lethargy, hypoglycemia - observe for irritability, tremors associated with hypocalcemia - administer ordered IV glucose, Ca, fluid replacements - provide ordered gavage, TPN
		RATIONALE: *The stress of surgery and the precipitating condition may increase nutritional requirements, yet limit options for adequate calorie/nutrient intake.*

NURSING DIAGNOSES	OUTCOME CRITERIA	INTERVENTIONS
4 High Risk for Altered Parenting *r.t. anxiety, interruptions of bonding*	• Parents discuss anatomy of surgery, ask appropriate questions, verbalize realistic perceptions	• Explain, discuss anatomy of the surgery, expected course, treatment rationale; allow for time to listen to fears, concerns
	• Parents visit, touch, hold, soothe infant	• Encourage parents to visit as often as possible; allow them to touch, hold, feed as condition permits • Parents demonstrate required infant care techniques
		RATIONALE: *The stress of having a neonate go to surgery may tax the parents' coping beyond their limits of adequate functioning.*
5 High Risk for Infection *r.t. bacterial invasion of surgical site, nosocomial infection*	• Exhibits no redness, edema, purulent drainage around incision	• Inspect incisional area for evidence of infection q2-4h prn after initial dressing change by surgeon
	• Displays no s/s of inflammation around insertion site of any chest or other tubes	• Inspect tube, drainage sites for signs of infection: redness, edema, drainage
	• Shows normal, stable axillary temperature	• Monitor axillary temperature qh until stable, then q2-4h
	• Shows normal WBC and differential	• Evaluate WBC, differential for evidence of infection responses

	• Shows negative cultures	• Collect cultures as ordered; evaluate results; report positive cultures
		
		• Protect infant from bacterial exposure
		  - maintain strict hand-washing techniques, universal precautions
		  - use sterile techniques for dressing changes, wound care, irrigations

		RATIONALE: *Sick neonates are at high risk for infection due to their poor immunological response.*

GENERAL

NURSING DIAGNOSES	OUTCOME CRITERIA	INTERVENTIONS
6 Pain *r.t. surgical incision, surgery, restriction of movement* *(Refer to "Pain Management" care plan)*	• Is free of s/s of uncontrolled pain - no extended agitation - consolable	• Monitor, manage pain; assess for s/s of pain qh - note agitation, increased HR or BP - provide comfort measures, quiet environment, positioning - administer analgesics per orders; assess effects, side effects **RATIONALE:** *Minimizing pain decreases potential for physiologic compromise due to distress/irritability.*

> **OTHER LESS COMMON NURSING DIAGNOSES:** *Ineffective Airway Clearance; Impaired Gas Exchange; High Risk for Altered Body Temperature; Altered Urinary Elimination; Impaired Skin Integrity; Sleep Pattern Disturbance; Activity Intolerance*

ESSENTIAL DISCHARGE CRITERIA

- Maintains balanced I&O
- Exhibits no respiratory distress, on room air
- Takes/retains 90% of feedings, with 20-30 g (0.7-1.05 oz) weight gain/day

- Parents demonstrate required post-op care techniques and express confidence in their won competencies
- Parents are able to comfort, console, and soothe infant

MEDICAL NURSING

CONTENTS

Intracranial Pressure, Increased
Juvenile Rheumatoid Arthritis
Leukemia
Meningitis
Meningomyelocele, Repaired (Older Child)
Near-SIDS Event (Sudden Infant Death Syndrome)
Nephrotic Syndrome
Neuroblastoma
Osteomyelitis
Pneumonia
Poisoning
Quadriplegia, Spinal Cord Injury
Respiratory Distress
Reye Syndrome
Seizure Disorders
Sickle Cell Disease
Systemic Lupus Erythematosus
Tuberculosis
Ulcerative Colitis
Wilms' Tumor

ABUSE/NEGLECT

NURSING DIAGNOSES	OUTCOME CRITERIA	INTERVENTIONS
1 High Risk for Injury *r.t. history of abuse, presence of household hazards*	• Experiences no further injuries	• Report injuries or suspected injuries to appropriate authorities • Refer family to child protective services assistance according to family's perceived need • Monitor family with respect to the likelihood of future injury to child or any siblings
	• Parents express perceived needs for help	• Refer family to protective services assistance according to family's perceived need • Monitor parental cooperation in following through with family therapy • Note any improvements in parent-child interaction • Discuss with the parents the commitment to learn and practice nonviolent coping strategies
		RATIONALE: *Acknowledgment of improved relations provides positive feedback and encourages continuation of treatment plan.*
2 Altered Growth and Development *r.t. inadequate caretaking, dysfunctional interaction*	• Exhibits normal growth and development patterns	• Assess child's developmental skills and physical, cognitive, and affective behaviors • Note areas of child's delayed development
	• Parents and child display adaptive changes in their interactions	• Be sure child has primary nurse • Demonstrate acceptance of child; provide nurturing interaction and consistent expectations • Provide age-appropriate stimulation • Provide consistent responses to child and affirm positive behaviors • Incorporate behavior modification to foster positive behavior • Refer family to community and professional resources for continued support

MEDICAL

43

NURSING DIAGNOSES	OUTCOME CRITERIA	INTERVENTIONS
		• Suggest the use of age-appropriate child care facilities to provide parents' "time out" and stimulation for child
		RATIONALE: *For development to progress, the child must be stimulated and be in a nurturing environment. Learning new behaviors and ways to cope with stress is difficult and requires long-term support and assistance.*
3 Self-Esteem Disturbance *r.t. emotional abuse, unmet basic needs*	• Displays self confidence - tries new skills - interacts with peers	• Observe and note child's behavior and interaction with peers • Provide time and safe environment for child to express feelings • Discuss appropriate peer interaction; clarify when aggression is appropriate and when it is not • Support the submissive child in gradual interactions with peers • Provide positive feedback • Observe child's response to questions about injuries • Observe child's reaction to hospital environment to identify unmet needs • Provide age-appropriate teaching and involve child in designing treatment plan • Encourage child to talk about positive experiences and happy times with parent • Acknowledge child's feelings for parent and validate the importance of parental care
	• Parents support/affirm child's abilities	• Involve parent in learning and giving support to child
		RATIONALE: *An abused child is at risk for developing a negative sense of self. It is essential to help the child begin to resolve feelings of ambiguity toward parent and to assist in the development of trust.*

NURSING DIAGNOSES	OUTCOME CRITERIA	INTERVENTIONS

4 Ineffective Family Coping
 	
r.t. emotional conflicts, highly ambivalent family relationships, situational crises
	• Parents cope/adapt to stress
	  - demonstrate appropriate use of resources
	  - use new behaviors that enhance ability to cope with stressors
		• Determine if child is in immediate danger; initiate protection; notify authorities
		• Assess parents' usual pattern of coping, i.e., whether parents show tendency to use force, power, or violence
		• Discuss use of community resources and family therapy
		• Discuss parents' perception of personal ability to control emotions such as anger
		• Encourage parent to describe events, behaviors, or situations that present coping difficulties
		• Have parent list stressors
		• Offer ways for parent to facilitate coping (time outs, counting to 100, planning ahead to avoid certain events)
		• Discuss plan with multidisciplinary team

		RATIONALE: *Parental participation in identification of coping strategies will enhance cooperation. Parents benefit from various coping strategy suggestions, none of which use force.*

5 Knowledge Deficit
 	
r.t. cognitive limitations with inability to state normal process of child's growth and development; unrealistic parental self-expectations
	• Parents demonstrate cognition of child's growth and development
	  - express realistic perceptions of child's abilities
	  - express expectations of the child's skills and behaviors that are age-appropriate
		• Determine the knowledge base of the parent
		• Review the aspects of normal growth and development
		• Support positive parenting behaviors and development of nuturing behaviors
		• Encourage parent to discuss personal perceptions of a child's behavior and document any misconceptions
		• Acknowledge the parent's frustration regarding changes that occur as child develops
		• Help parent identify positive feedback from child

MEDICAL

ABUSE/NEGLECT

NURSING DIAGNOSES	OUTCOME CRITERIA	INTERVENTIONS
		• Provide clarification and anticipatory guidance regarding the behavior that the parent finds difficult
		• Act as a role model for parent by having appropriate, positive interaction with child
		• Demonstrate ways for the parent to promote development of the child through stimulating play and realistic expectations
		• Provide resources for parent to obtain additional information

RATIONALE: *The ability to express empathy will foster open communication. Keeping expectations reasonable facilitates cooperation.*

OTHER LESS COMMON NURSING DIAGNOSES: *Altered Family Processes*

ESSENTIAL DISCHARGE CRITERIA

- Sustains no further injury
- Is confident; tries new skills; interacts with staff, family, peers
- Parents demonstrate appropriate use of resources

- Parents describe realistic perceptions of child's abilities
- Parents demonstrate positive parent-child interaction
- Child returns to an environment verified as safe

46

APLASTIC ANEMIA

NURSING DIAGNOSES	OUTCOME CRITERIA	INTERVENTIONS

1 Altered Tissue Perfusion
 	
r.t. insufficient RBCs for O_2 transport
	• Shows improved tissue perfusion
	  - adequate urine output
	  - strong peripheral pulses
	  - capillary refill < 3 sec
	  - pulse, BP, respirations WNL
		• Assess pulse, respirations, peripheral pulses and capillary refill q2-4h
		
		• Monitor for s/s of hemorrhage
		  - VS, bleeding sites, skin color, weakness, and LOC
		
		• Administer and monitor response to blood products
		  - Hct and Hb lab values
		  - report any abnormalities

		RATIONALE: *Early detection and management prevent further hypoxemia of peripheral tissues.*
2 Anxiety *r.t. perceived threat from diagnostic and treatment procedures*	• Demonstrates understanding of procedures	• Provide age-appropriate education to child about procedures and sensations • Establish a trusting relationship
	• Displays minimal anxiety levels	• Assess current anxiety levels of child and family • Assign consistent hospital caregivers • Provide familiar environment (toys, parents) • Maintain home routines and rituals

	• Parents participate in care	• Educate family about care requirements
		  - child's condition and procedures
		  - monitoring for s/s of infection and bleeding
		  - measures to prevent infection
		  - community support systems for long-term adaptation (school integration, parent, child, sibling, and family groups)

	• Parent/child cooperate with care	• Provide a safe environment for the child and family to express anxiety and feelings surrounding procedures • Encourage participation of primary caregiver
		RATIONALE: *Reduction of anxiety promotes cooperation and improves health outcomes.*

MEDICAL

APLASTIC ANEMIA

NURSING DIAGNOSES	OUTCOME CRITERIA	INTERVENTIONS
3 Altered Nutrition: Less than body requirements *r.t. reported inadequate iron intake, knowledge deficit regarding iron-rich foods*	• Takes increased dietary iron	• Assess and promote adequate nutritional intake • Explore family eating habits • Monitor child's intake • Administer iron as ordered • Collaborate with dietitian in developing a diet plan that considers eating habits, nutritional needs, financial, and environmental resources • Instruct family and child on appropriate nutritional intake
	• Family/child demonstrate knowledge of iron-rich foods	• Educate child, family about increasing dietary iron and importance of long-term iron therapy
		RATIONALE: *Increasing iron intake promotes production of blood components and helps improve the child's physical condition.*
4 High Risk for Activity Intolerance *r.t. generalized weakness*	• Exhibits tolerance for increased activity - VS WNL with increased activity - cooperates with increased activities	• Assess current desired activity levels • Monitor pulse, BP, and RR with activity and rest • Provide periods of physical activity followed by uninterrupted rest • Gradually increase activity levels and length of time • Provide quiet play activities for diversion • Coordinate activities to occur during periods of greatest energy • Administer O_2 as ordered
	• Parents participate in providing paced activity and evaluating activity tolerance	• Encourage family to participate in gradual increase in child's activities • Educate family and child to recognize signs of activity intolerance and appropriate interventions

NURSING DIAGNOSES	OUTCOME CRITERIA	INTERVENTIONS
	• Participates in age-appropriate play	• Collaborate with Child Life specialist for appropriate activities (physical and at rest)
		• Coordinate continuation of plan at home and school

RATIONALE: *Pacing improves activity tolerance. Age-appropriate play activities promote growth and development.*

OTHER LESS COMMON NURSING DIAGNOSES: *High Risk for Injury (internal, external); High Risk for Infection; Altered Growth and Development*

ESSENTIAL DISCHARGE CRITERIA

- Has normal respiratory and pulse rate
- Shows O_2 saturation WNL
- Has strong peripheral pulses, good capillary refill

- VS remain stable with increased activity
- Child/family select and plan iron-rich foods for child's home menu

MEDICAL

ASTHMA, BRONCHIOLITIS

NURSING DIAGNOSES	OUTCOME CRITERIA	INTERVENTIONS
1 Impaired Gas Exchange *r.t. ventilation perfusion imbalance*	• Exhibits balanced ventilation perfusion - ABGs WNL - VS WNL - displays age-appropriate behavior	• Monitor ABGs for decreased PCO_2 and pH, and increased PCO_2 levels; utilize pulse oximetry and/or transcutaneous PCO_2 monitoring
	• Presents no adverse effects	• Check VS qh during initial treatment, then q2-4h • Assess RR qh (1 full min); assess for presence of dyspnea, retractions, nasal flaring, apnea • Assess for changes in LOC, activity, signs of irritability and/or restlessness • Elevate child's head to improve air exchange • Administer O_2 via appropriate measure (hood, tent, cannula, mask) - adjust O_2 according to ABGs and physician's orders • Administer bronchodilators, corticosteroids as ordered; assess for side effects: nausea, vomiting, restlessness, seizures, coma
		RATIONALE: *Early identification of respiratory failure allows for early intervention.*
2 Ineffective Airway Clearance *r.t. tracheobronchial infection, obstruction, secretions*	• Exhibits normal RR, depth, and ease - no adventitious breath sounds - diminishing cough - diminishing secretions - skin color is normal	• Assess RR, depth, and ease, initially q30min then q1-2h (count respirations for 1 full min) • Assess breath sounds by auscultation q1-2h • Assess cough q1-2h (moist, harsh, croupy) • Assess color and consistency of secretions and ability to expectorate q1-2h • Assess skin color changes and duration; check mucus membranes, nail beds q1-2h • Elevate HOB or hold infant in upright position

NURSING DIAGNOSES	OUTCOME CRITERIA	INTERVENTIONS
		• Reposition child q2h
		• Provide cool mist vaporizer or mist tent
		RATIONALE: *These measures will help prevent airway obstruction and possible respiratory failure and promote mobilization of secretions.*
3 High Risk for Fluid Volume Deficit *r.t. insufficient intake secondary to dyspnea and malaise, insensible water loss from tachypnea*	• Shows normal fluid and electrolyte balance	• Monitor I&O q8h (weigh diapers for infants) • Monitor urinary sp. gr. q8h • Weigh daily (same scale, naked, before breakfast) • Monitor serum electrolytes, BUN, creatinine, Hb, Hct

	• Shows good hydration
	  - normal fontanel and eye tension
	  - produces tears
	  - moist mucous membranes
	  - good skin turgor
	  - normal VS
		• Administer acetaminophen or pediatric ibuprofen if temp > 38° C (100.4° F) as orderd
		• Assess for sunken fontanel, sunken eyes, dry mucous membranes, absence of tears, poor skin turgor q4h
		• Assess for changes in VS (tachycardia)
		• Increase PO fluids when condition improves
		• Feed slowly, with frequent rest periods
		• Assess likes and dislikes; provide favorites as permitted and tolerated
		• Administer IV fluids as ordered; monitor IV rate hourly; check site patency
		• Explain to parents and child amount of fluid needed and rationale based on illness

		RATIONALE: *Early detection of s/s of dehydration produces prompt management and prevents serious consequences related to fluid deficit and electrolyte imbalance.*

MEDICAL

NURSING DIAGNOSES	OUTCOME CRITERIA	INTERVENTIONS
4 Fatigue *r.t. respiratory effort*	• Shows increased endurance and improved respiratory function	• Assess for extreme weakness and fatigue, change in LOC or behavior • Disturb infant or child only when necessary • Schedule rest periods in a quiet and comfortable environment • Allow quiet play with familiar toy while maintaining bedrest • Inform parents of measures to take to prevent fatigue and of reason to conserve energy

RATIONALE: *These measures help the patient to breathe efficiently and reduce or minimize fatigue.*

OTHER LESS COMMON NURSING DIAGNOSES: Altered Nutrition: Less than body requirements; Hyperthermia; Anxiety; Knowledge Deficit; Activity Intolerance

ESSENTIAL DISCHARGE CRITERIA

• Exhibits RR and effort WNL

• Maintains thin, clear secretions that can be mobilized or removed from airway via nasal bulb suctioning

• Maintains adequate hydration status

• Parent/child identifies s/s to be reported for follow-up treatment

AUTONOMIC DYSREFLEXIA

NURSING DIAGNOSES	OUTCOME CRITERIA	INTERVENTIONS
1 High Risk for Injury (internal) *r.t. hypertension associated with spinal cord injuries above T-5*	• Achieves, maintains stable VS - pulse increasing to WNL	• Monitor BP, VS q3-5min during crisis, then q15-30min, then as ordered

	• Is free of s/s of sympathetic hyperactivity
	  - sweating
	  - gooseflesh
	  - nausea
	  - seizure activity
	  - headache
		• Monitor for s/s of hyperactive sympathetic system q2-4h

	• Experiences prompt reversal of symptoms (by 8h post admission)	• Prevent, manage symptoms
		  - elevate HOB
		  - assess for s/s of causes (distended bladder, bowel dilation or overdistention, pressure points)
		  - initiate seizure precautions, including O2 and suction at bedside

		RATIONALE: *Constant monitoring, for stabilizing hypertension provides data for assessing success of ongoing management strategies.*
2 Altered Urinary Elimination *r.t. sensory and neuromuscular impairment*	• Shows urinary output WNL for age, weight	• Monitor urinary output qh during acute phase

	• Achieves normal urinary output
	  - no retention
	  - no incontinence
	  - no frequency
	  - no hesitancy or dysuria
		• Manage urinary alterations per orders, unit protocol
		  - monitor for urinary retention
		  - incontinence (in children with injuries to T-5 or above)
		  - assess urinary function after catheter removal
		  - expect potential for intermittent I&O catheter, Credé maneuver of bladder
		  - catheterize using anesthetic, noting amount, color, consistency; assess BP when finished
		  - if Foley in place and clogged: unkink, drain bag; obtain orders to gently irrigate or insert new catheter

		RATIONALE: *Assessing, monitoring, and prompt management of urinary retention is important to prevent overdistention of bladder.*

MEDICAL

NURSING DIAGNOSES	OUTCOME CRITERIA	INTERVENTIONS
3 Constipation *r.t. neuromuscular damage*	• Shows no mass of hard stool on palpation	• Perform rectal exam if dilation not cause; if rectal mass present, remove using anesthetic ointment; assess BP
	• Experiences stool continence; has bowel pattern established	• Manage bowel program - stop any bowel dilation if on bowel program - assess BP - inspect abdomen for distention (may require NG tube) - maintain bowel routine
		RATIONALE: *Because of the neuromuscular damage, constipation must be carefully managed. A consistent, regular bowel regimen is necessary.*
4 High Risk for Impaired Skin Integrity *r.t. altered sensory perception*	• Shows no evidence of pressure points, including feet, toes	• Monitor, manage skin care - inspect all pressure areas q2h - inspect skin for redness, injury, pallor q2h - change position, remove any potential pressures q2h - provide alternating pressure, eggcrate mattress, sheepskin
	• Parents/child describe how to prevent future pressure areas	• Describe, demonstrate skin care
		RATIONALE: *Meticulous monitoring and management of skin condition is necessary because of neuromuscular and sensory impairment. Changing position and avoiding pressure points prevent skin breakdown.*
5 Knowledge Deficit *r.t. disease process, home care, follow-up medical supervision*	• Parents/child discuss physiology of disease process, rationale for treatment	• Teach parent/child all interventions and their rationale as outlined in care plan
	• Parents/child verbalize knowledge of s/s of autonomic crisis: headache, elevated BP, slow pulse, gooseflesh, sweating, skin blotching above T-5, nasal congestion, nausea	• Describe s/s of autonomic crisis

NURSING DIAGNOSES	OUTCOME CRITERIA	INTERVENTIONS
	• Parents demonstrate required care - preventative procedures - emergency interventions	• Instruct parents to perform preventative, emergency procedures • Provide written copy of all instructions • Provide home care supervision to assist with preventative regime as indicated
	• Parents possess phone numbers of emergency medical help in event of crisis	• Provide emergency phone numbers
	• Parents verbalize knowledge of follow-up appointments	• Verify knowledge of follow-up appointments
		RATIONALE: *Knowledgeable, competent parents are likely to prevent or successfully manage crisis in future.*

MEDICAL

OTHER LESS COMMON NURSING DIAGNOSES: High Risk for Caregiver Role Strain

---

ESSENTIAL DISCHARGE CRITERIA

• Is normotensive

• Maintains normal urinary output, bowel routine

• Parents verbalize knowledge about disease process, treatment rationale, complications, s/s of crisis

• Parents demonstrate competence with crisis prevention and emergency procedures

• Parents verbalize knowledge of follow-up appointments and have phone numbers and location of nearest emergency services

BILIARY ATRESIA

NURSING DIAGNOSES	OUTCOME CRITERIA	INTERVENTIONS
1 Altered Nutrition: Less than body requirements *r.t. inability to digest fats*	• Maintains weight in the same percentile for age on standardized growth curve until surgical correction is complete	• Weigh daily
	• Displays no signs of vitamin deficiency - cracked lips	• For infant, diet including predigested fats (e.g., Tolorex) • Diet may include formula, such as Portagen or Pregestimil • For children other than infants, provide diet high in CHO and low in fat • Administer supplemental fat-soluble vitamins A, D, E, and K as ordered • Administer TPN or intralipids as ordered
	• Passes normal stools	• Monitor stool, pattern, frequency
	• Parents understand and are comfortable with the diet management plan	• Explain fat digestion; include parents in dietary planning
		RATIONALE: *Bile salts are required for absorption of dietary fats and fat-soluble vitamins. Medium-chain fatty acids and predigested formula can be digested without the need for bile. Children who evidence significant malabsorption problems may need TPN or intralipids.*
2 Anticipatory Grieving *r.t. uncertain prognosis and loss of "perfect baby"*	• Family members demonstrate support for each other through the grieving process	• Establish an open, honest, caring professional relationship • Encourage family to express perceptions and feelings of current situation so the grieving process can begin • Provide active listening in a quiet, private environment • Discuss and identify impact of anticipated loss • Keep family informed

NURSING DIAGNOSES	OUTCOME CRITERIA	INTERVENTIONS
		• Assist family in identifying its coping strengths and coping strategies that are effective
	• Family can identify its major support systems that will be mobilized to meet the family members' needs	• Assist the family in identifying and mobilizing support systems
	• Family demonstrates understanding of the disease process and treatment approaches	• Offer clarification of procedures, treatment, or plans for patient and family • Encourage parental and sibling participation in care of infant or child according to situation
		RATIONALE: *A trusting relationship between the nurse and family provides for a safe, supportive environment for the grieving process to begin. Helping the family to mobilize its resources by using its own strengths and coping strategies will empower the family.*
3 Altered Family Processes *r.t. child with chronic illness requiring frequent hospitalizations and clinic visits*	• Family demonstrates understanding of treatment regimen	• Encourage parent and sibling participation in patient's hospitalization, procedures, and plans for discharge
	• Family demonstrates that it can maintain and support functional family roles - participates in care - discusses family goals - plans and enacts normal life style behaviors	• Help family organize to continue usual family activities • Reinforce parents' knowledge and caretaking behaviors • Assist family in establishing realistic goals for short-term and long-term needs • Discuss with the family how the current situation affects family roles and possible changes that may be necessary • Reinforce family accomplishments

MEDICAL

NURSING DIAGNOSES	OUTCOME CRITERIA	INTERVENTIONS

RATIONALE: *Inclusion of all family members and positive reinforcement of family strengths empower the family to continue to work together in a healthy, functional fashion. Recognition that hospitalization is only one facet of the continuum of care of the chronically ill family member assures more appropriate and successful intervention.*

OTHER LESS COMMON NURSING DIAGNOSES: *High Risk for Impaired Skin Integrity; High Risk for Fluid Volume Deficit; Altered Health Maintenance; Altered Growth and Development; Altered Parenting; Knowledge Deficit; High Risk for Caregiver Role Strain*

ESSENTIAL DISCHARGE CRITERIA

- Maintains stable or increasing weight
- Parents demonstrate understanding of signs of cholangitis and other complications of biliary atresia
- Family members offer/provide mutual support

- Parents demonstrate proficiency in administering medications
- Parents demonstrate knowledge of diet therapy
- Parents/family participate in care, make plans, enact many normal life style roles and behaviors

NURSING DIAGNOSES	OUTCOME CRITERIA	INTERVENTIONS
1 Ineffective Breathing Pattern *r.t. neuromuscular impairment*	• Experiences support of airway and respiration - has RR, rhythm WNL - has normal chest expansion and skin color - has clear breath sounds - has normal tidal volume	• Monitor effectiveness of breathing pattern: rate, rhythm, breath sounds, and tidal volume • Perform pulmonary toilet q4h and suction q4h and prn • Anticipate need for mechanical ventilatory support
	• Exhibits gag reflex	• Monitor gag reflex and swallow; keep NPO if absent • Position on side, prone, or with head elevated
	• Has normal ABGs	• Assess ABGs, pulse oximetry
		RATIONALE: *Constant monitoring of respiratory function results in effective management of ventilation, which, in turn, prevents airway obstruction, atelectasis, and pneumonia.*
2 Impaired Swallowing *r.t. neuromuscular impairment*	• Shows improvement in swallowing - exhibits protective reflexes (gag and cough) - has strong suck with coordinated swallow	• Monitor gag/cough reflex while suctioning mouth; if absent, do not feed orally • Monitor swallow by observing pooling of oral secretions or drooling • Position on side, prone, or with head elevated • Confirm feeding tube placement; check residual volume (prior to NG/OG feeding) • Position on right side with head slightly elevated (during and after NG/OG feedings)
		RATIONALE: *Assessment of the infant's ability to protect airway prevents aspiration. Supportive positioning and feeding lessen chance of regurgitation or aspiration.*

MEDICAL

NURSING DIAGNOSES	OUTCOME CRITERIA	INTERVENTIONS
3 Colonic Constipation *r.t. neuromuscular impairment, inadequate physical activity*	• Maintains bowel function	• Monitor frequency and consistency of stools • Increase intake of fluids • Perform gentle rectal (thermometer) stimulation • Administer stool softeners if ordered
		RATIONALE: *A soft stool is easier to pass. Taking rectal temperature may relax the sphincter to allow the stool to pass.*
4 Altered Nutrition: Less than body requirements *r.t. neuromuscular impairment, inability to nipple-feed/eat*	• Exhibits evidence of adequate nutritional intake - normalizing body weight - balanced I&O - good skin turgor, moist mucous membranes - normal urinary sp. gr. - normal serum electrolytes	• Monitor weight daily using same scale, same time of day • Maintain accurate I&O • Assess for dehydration: skin turgor, urine sp. gr., serum electrolytes, and mucous membranes
	• Takes, retains feedings	• Monitor gag reflex and swallow; if weak or absent, do not feed orally • Administer feedings as ordered • Confirm tube placement and check residual volume (prior to NG feeding) • Position on right side with head slightly elevated (during and after NG feeding)
		RATIONALE: *Adequate calories and water maintain weight and organ function. Adequate nutrition supports healing and growth. Small, continuous feeds are less likely to cause regurgitation and aspiration.*

NURSING DIAGNOSES	OUTCOME CRITERIA	INTERVENTIONS
5 Urinary Retention *r.t. neuromuscular impairment*	• Shows no evidence of urinary retention	• Monitor volume of urine (minimum 1-3mL/kg/h) • Palpate for bladder fullness q4h • If full, perform gentle Credé maneuver of bladder to facilitate emptying
	• Shows normal urinary sp. gr.	• Monitor sp. gr. q8h and prn

RATIONALE: *Monitoring and managing urinary residual prevent urinary tract infections secondary to stasis.*

OTHER LESS COMMON NURSING DIAGNOSES:
High Risk for Aspiration; Fatigue; Caregiver Role Strain; Knowledge Deficit

---

ESSENTIAL DISCHARGE CRITERIA

• Maintains and protects airway

• Takes adequate calories for growth

• Shows normal bowel function

• Urinary output is WNL

MEDICAL

BRAIN TUMOR

NURSING DIAGNOSES	OUTCOME CRITERIA	INTERVENTIONS
1 Altered Thought Processes *r.t. altered circulation or destruction of brain tissue*	• Reveals no s/s of abnormal neurological status • Shows stable, normal VS/BP	• VS/BP q2h and prn; note any trends (increasing HR, decreasing RR, widening pulse pressure)

	• Shows evidence of alertness and orientation
	  - no personality changes
	  - motor strength equal in all extremities
	  - gait steady
	  - PERL
	  - no visual disturbances
	  - speech clear
	  - olfactory intact
	  - no seizure activity
		• Check neurological signs q2h and prn
		  - note any abnormal behavior
		  - monitor ability to follow commands
		  - assess and document strength and equality of grip
		  - assess and document pupillary size, shape, response to light, ability to track in all directions
		  - note facial symmetry, any drooling, inability to maintain tongue in mouth
		  - document patient's verbalization of any unusual odors
		  - document any seizure activity noting time, duration, and body involvement
		  - notify physician of any changes

		RATIONALE: *Regular monitoring of neurological signs allows early detection of any neurological deterioration.*
2 High Risk for Injury (external) *r.t. altered neurological status*	• Sustains no injuries	• Keep bed in low position • Raise side rails up when patient is asleep and prn • Pad rails • Provide chair with arms • Place call light within reach of patient • Ensure that nursing personnel are in attendance when patient is up in chair or ambulating • Remove any sharp, potentially harmful objects • Include parents in monitoring safety precautions • Avoid or space required nursing activities that increase intracranial pressure
		RATIONALE: *Using safety precautions helps prevent injury to the patient.*

NURSING DIAGNOSES	OUTCOME CRITERIA	INTERVENTIONS

3 Pain
r.t. pressure from tumor, edema, or surgery
	• Verbalizes/displays freedom from headache
	  - relaxed body posture and facial expressions
		• Perform a comprehensive assessment of pain, utilizing age-appropriate pediatric pain assessment tools; document q2-4h
		
		• Provide pain relief measures, monitoring and documenting effectiveness
		  - administer ordered analgesics and related medications on a schedule to prevent breakthrough pain if possible
		  - reduce or eliminate factors that precipitate or increase pain experience (room temperature, lighting, noise, fear)
		  - elevate HOB unless contraindicated
		  - give emotional/physical support during painful periods

RATIONALE: *Minimizing/alleviating pain will minimize increased intracranial pressure.*

MEDICAL

OTHER LESS COMMON NURSING DIAGNOSES:
Fear; Sensory/Perceptual Alteration; Anticipatory Grieving; Anxiety

ESSENTIAL DISCHARGE CRITERIA

• Exhibits evidence of alertness and orientation

• Verbalizes/displays freedom from pain

• Demonstrates ability to perform ADLs

• Parents verbalize plan for follow-up and list s/s reportable to PCP

CANCER

See Nursing Care Plan "Chemotherapy"

1 Knowledge Deficit

r.t. diagnosis and associated treatments

- Parents verbalize knowledge of diagnosis, treatment, and major precautions

- Facilitate discussion of diagnosis/treatments and prognosis with family and physician
- Encourage family to verbalize questions and concerns
- Discuss precautions needed for self/child and rationale, e.g., protective isolation, limited visitors

RATIONALE: *Thorough understanding of the diagnosis is necessary for compliance with treatment regimen.*

2 Powerlessness

r.t. diagnosis, hospitalization, treatment

- Parent/child identify things he/she can control

- Encourage child and parents to assist in planning care (what time to bathe, pain medication before uncomfortable procedures, food and fluid preferences); document in plan of care
- Keep items child needs within reach
- Allow child to take control of as many ADLs as possible
- Praise accomplishments

- Family/child express feelings and concerns, ask questions, seek clarification

- Encourage verbalization of concern through active listening
- Provide family/child with oncology information that pertains to their diagnosis
- Notify social worker, chaplain, play therapist, and psychologist of child's admission
- Explain all procedures to the child before they occur
- Use play therapy to encourage expressions of feelings and explain procedures

RATIONALE: *Understanding of what is going on gives some control and decreases anxiety.*

> **OTHER LESS COMMON NURSING DIAGNOSES:**
> *Altered Protection; Body Image Disturbance; Spiritual Distress; Fear*

ESSENTIAL DISCHARGE CRITERIA

- Family/child describe diagnosis and treatment

- Family/child have printed information about local support groups, service agencies

- Family/child actively participate in planning daily activities

- Parent/child verbalize s/s reportable to PCP, plan follow-up visits

MEDICAL

CEREBRAL PALSY

NURSING DIAGNOSES	OUTCOME CRITERIA	INTERVENTIONS
1 Impaired Physical Mobility *r.t. neuromuscular impairment*	• Achieves mobility within limits of disability	• Provide appropriate assistive devices: braces, wheelchairs, special equipment, etc. • Perform ROM, repositioning in bed q2h if on bedrest • Educate family to assist with and perform appropriate exercises to increase mobility • Encourage mobility to child's level through the use of play and/or special interest • Seek consultation: physical therapy, rehabilitation therapy, etc.
		RATIONALE: *Consistent attention to various forms of mobility prevents further immobility and deterioration of child's physical structure.*
2 High Risk for Injury (external) *r.t. neuromuscular and cerebral impairment*	• Sustains no further physical injury	• Provide a safe environment, free from hazards - side rails up on beds and cribs, bubble top crib - extraneous equipment and toys cleared away - clean, dry floors - dependable, safe equipment/assistive devices • Allow for adequate rest times • Provide age-appropriate as well as disability-appropriate toys • Arrange for caregiver to be present during self-care activities to prevent accidents (choking, falling)
		RATIONALE: *Providing protection through a safe environment prevents injury to the child.*

NURSING DIAGNOSES	OUTCOME CRITERIA	INTERVENTIONS
3 Self-Care Deficits (bathing/ hygiene, dressing/ grooming, feeding, toileting) *r.t. physical component of this chronic disability*	• Performs activities of self-care appropriate with physical capabilities	• Include child in planning own self-care activities, e.g., times of bath, menu planning • Remain patient, allowing child enough time to complete self-care tasks • Provide assistive devices enabling child to begin/complete tasks • Encourage to partake in any part of self-care • Instruct parents on techniques that may help with self-care, e.g. jaw control during feeding, toilet training
		RATIONALE: *Facilitating self-care fosters the child's sense of independence and control and prevents regression of self-care activities as a result of hospitalization.*
4 Total Incontinence *r.t. neouromuscular impairment*	• Stools and voids alone or with assistance, as appropriate	• Set up surroundings so that it is easy for child to void/stool on own • Become knowledgeable of child's patterns at home and adapt hospital schedule accordingly • Inquire q2h as to child's disposition: offer bedpan, help to bathroom • Initiate sterile intermittent catheterization as needed • Teach intermittent self-catheterization when appropriate
		RATIONALE: *When the child maintains a routine voiding/stooling schedule, he/she avoids incontinence and embarrassment and promotes regularity.*

MEDICAL

NURSING DIAGNOSES	OUTCOME CRITERIA	INTERVENTIONS

5 Fatigue
r.t. interrupted sleep and increased expended energy
	• Is free of s/s of chronic fatigue
	  - well rested
	  - alert
	  - good appetite
		• Observe for signs of fatigue
		  - lethargy
		  - anorexia
		  - listlessness
		  - activity intolerance
		• Keep routine schedule (as close to home schedule as possible); minimize interruptions
		• Cluster and pace care activities to allow for extended rest periods and sleep

	• Achieves, maintains normal weight	• Weigh daily • Provide adequate nutrition and calories to maintain daily energy requirements (consult nutritionist prn)
		RATIONALE: *Providing adequate rest reduces energy demands, and nutrition provides more energy to meet metabolic requirements. Minimizing chronic fatigue fosters normal physical and social growth and development.*

6 Impaired Verbal Communication
r.t. inability to articulate spoken words and/or hearing loss due to cerebral damage
	• Is able to communicate needs and can understand communication directed at him/her
	  - decreasing displays of frustration
	  - responds appropriately to questions, requests
		• Involve speech therapist
		• Allow extra time for giving care to ensure successful communication
		• Use pictures, items, gestures to aid in communication as needed (posters, typewriters, computers, sign language)

		RATIONALE: *With adequate communication, the child has his/her needs met and experiences decreased frustration and social isolation.*

NURSING DIAGNOSES	OUTCOME CRITERIA	INTERVENTIONS
7 Altered Family Processes *r.t. chronic disability of child*	• Family participates in care of child in an effective, healthy manner, while still maintaining balance in the family structure	• Include parents in planning and implementing hospital care, respecting their experience, expertise • Continue to educate family about CP and child's condition

	• Parents express concerns, ask questions, make plans for home care	• Provide time for family to express feelings, concerns
		
		• Involve parents in active planning for home care
		
		• Obtain support for family
		  - support groups, counseling as needed
		  - home care follow-up
		  - respite care
		  - rehabilitation and physical therapy as part of home care when appropriate
		  - coordination of multidisciplinary team
		  - suggest family members take time for themselves and maintain all relationships in family; refer to respite program

RATIONALE: *Through support, knowledge, self-care, and balance of the family structure, the child with CP will receive optimal care.*

OTHER LESS COMMON NURSING DIAGNOSES: *High Risk for Caregiver Role Strain; Altered Nutrition: Less than body requirements; High Risk for Impaired Skin Integrity; Body Image Disturbance; Self-Esteem Disturbance*

ESSENTIAL DISCHARGE CRITERIA

• Takes adequate diet with weight maintenance or appropriate gain/loss

• Has warm, dry, intact skin

• Performs ADL to limit of ability; participates in play activity to limit of ability

• Takes adequate sleep/rest periods

• Parents demonstrate safe care of child, verbalizing knowledge of medications and follow-up appointments

MEDICAL

CHEMICAL ADDICTION/WITHDRAWAL, INFANT

NURSING DIAGNOSES	OUTCOME CRITERIA	INTERVENTIONS

1 Altered Nutrition: Less than body requirements
 	
r.t. feeding problems, uncoordinated or ineffective sucking and swallowing and breathing, diarrhea, vomiting, colic
	• Maintains optimal nutritional status
	  - gains weight WNL
	  - has balanced I&O
		• Monitor and record nutritional intake based on calories and volume
		• Record daily weights
		• Monitor fluid and electrolyte status
		• Monitor daily intake and output

	• Coordinates suck, swallow, breathing	• Assess suck, swallow, breathing coordination
	• Is able to nipple adequate calories for growth	• Provide fortified formula; supplement breast milk as needed • Initiate gavage feedings when necessary • Give small frequent feedings • Minimize sensory stimuli during feedings • Use pacifier to satisfy non-nutritional sucking needs
	• Parents participate in feeding, demonstrate effective feeding techniques	• Teach parents/caregivers strategies for effective feedings
		RATIONALE: *Minimize feeding problems and prevent complications related to poor nutritional status.*

2 Sleep Pattern Disturbance
 	
r.t. effects of illicit drugs or medication
	• Sleeps, naps at age-appropriate intervals	• Monitor infant's sleep pattern
		• Allow for uninterrupted periods of sleep
		• Use calming techniques
		  - swaddling
		  - skin-to-skin contact
		  - vertical rocking
		  - use of front pack
		• Provide a dark, quiet environment

		RATIONALE: *Promote adequate rest to the infant. Environmental interventions may impact sleep patterns as well as changes in state-related behavior such as hyperirritability.*

NURSING DIAGNOSES	OUTCOME CRITERIA	INTERVENTIONS
3 High Risk for Injury (external) *r.t. increased hyperirritability and potential for seizure activity*	• Displays decreasing irritability - absence of seizure activity - no prolonged crying - relaxed body movements, facial expressions	• Reduce stimuli in nursery environment • Administer appropriate medications as ordered
	• Has timely recognition and treatment of seizure activity	• Keep O$_2$ available • Keep suction set up
	• Parents participate in calming and protecting infant	• Teach parents about safety measures and strategies to reduce irritability - swaddle infant when possible - rock vertically, not horizontally (use baby swings) - provide soft, quiet toys
		RATIONALE: *Calming measures reduce irritating stimuli. Protection reduces risk of seizure-related injury.*
4 Diarrhea *r.t. effects of withdrawal, increased peristalsis secondary to hyperirritability*	• Achieves, maintains stooling and consistency WNL - no more than 4-6 stools/day - no liquid stools	• Observe and record number and consistency of stools each day • Assess abdomen; note bowel sounds • Observe skin turgor • Test stools: Hematest, Clinatest
	• Shows balanced I&O	• Monitor and record intake and output • Monitor serum electrolytes
	• Parents discuss and affirm need to monitor, seek help for persistent diarrhea	• Teach parents/caregivers to seek medical attention if diarrhea persists for more than 24h • Teach parents the signs of dehydration
		RATIONALE: *Monitoring and managing gastric hyperirritability prevent complications related to diarrhea.*

MEDICAL

NURSING DIAGNOSES	OUTCOME CRITERIA	INTERVENTIONS
5 High Risk for Impaired Skin Integrity *r.t. GI disturbance (diarrhea) or friction rubs (due to hyperactivity)*	• Is free of excoriation or other skin breakdown - no breaks in skin - no redness, excoriation	• Observe and record skin condition q4h • Refrain from the use of tape when possible • Use mild soap and water • Change diapers immediately after each elimination - use cloth diapers - apply protective ointment as needed • Use sheepskin in crib or isolette • Place permeable, transparent dressings over friction rub areas - elbows - knees - chin
		RATIONALE: *Use of mild soap prevents allergic skin reaction. Frequent diapering prevents chemical skin burns from excretions. Protective ointments minimize contact between skin and irritants. Sheepskin reduces pressure areas.*
6 Altered Growth and Development *r.t. effects of maternal drug use, neurological impairment, decreased attentiveness to environmental stimuli*	• Shows growth and development patterns within normal limits - achieves optimal neurological function - attention deficits decreased - in contact with community resources	• Assess growth and development patterns of infant • Incorporate age-appropriate activities into the plan of care • Teach parents/caregivers about - normal patterns of growth and development - activities that support growth and development - behavior modification techniques - how to handle regressive behavior - community resources
		RATIONALE: *These measures foster the child's maximum potential growth and development.*

NURSING DIAGNOSES	OUTCOME CRITERIA	INTERVENTIONS

7 Altered Parenting
 	
r.t. substance abuse, impairment or lack of attachment behaviors, inadequate support systems
	• Parents display bonding behaviors
	  - provide personal care of infant (dress, diaper, feed)
	  - hold, touch, rock
	  - make eye contact with infant
	  - talk, croon to infant
		• Assess client's readiness to bond with infant
		
		• Provide early and repeated parent/infant contact
		
		• Encourage and reinforce parenting behavior
		
		• Document parent/child interaction
		
		• Encourage verbalization about perception of the child and feelings about parenting (fears, anger, frustrations)
		
		• Encourage parent(s) to room-in and assume total care for their child prior to discharge
		
		• Refer to support services and support groups as needed
		
		• Observe parent's understanding of the need for a nurturing environment

RATIONALE: *These measures foster the parents' understanding of the importance of a nurturing environment. Drug-exposed infants may be difficult to care for and therefore cause feelings of inadequacy and interrupted bonding between parents and infant.*

MEDICAL

OTHER LESS COMMON NURSING DIAGNOSES: *High Risk for Infection; Ineffective Airway Clearance; Sensory/Perceptual Alterations; High Risk for Caregiver Role Strain*

ESSENTIAL DISCHARGE CRITERIA

• Maintains age-appropriate weight gain

• Coordinates suck, swallow, and breathing reflexes

• Parents demonstrate effective care techniques (feeding, medicating, protecting, monitoring for diarrhea, weight loss, hyperirritability)

• Parents display bonding, comforting behaviors

CHEMICAL DEPENDENCY, ADOLESCENT

NURSING DIAGNOSES	OUTCOME CRITERIA	INTERVENTIONS
1 High Risk for Fluid Volume Deficit *r.t. vomiting, diarrhea, inability to tolerate oral fluids*	• Exhibits adequate fluid volume - balanced I&O - urinary sp. gr. WNL - HR/BP (specify acceptable range for patient) - no nausea, vomiting - moist mucous membranes; elastic skin recoil - presence of bowel sounds - no abdominal distention	• Monitor I&O q8h • Monitor urinary sp. gr. q void or as indicated • Assess VS q4h or as indicated • Inspect mucous membranes, skin turgor q4h • Assess for nausea, anorexia q4-8h • Assess bowel sounds, abdominal girth q2-4h or as indicated • Provide preferred fluids • Explain reason for high fluid intake • Discuss with patient/family need for fluids and graduation to solids as tolerated • Administer parenteral fluids as ordered • Administer prescribed medications designed to control or substitute for illicit drug or medication • Identify areas of probable noncompliance for special dietary counseling or referrals **RATIONALE:** *Early detection and prompt management of fluid deficit are essential to prevent dehydration which interferes with correction of primary medical diagnosis.*
2 Altered Nutrition: Less than body requirements *r.t. anorexia, diarrhea, hyperactivity, lethargy associated with effects of illicit drugs or medications*	• Is able to take required calories - receives, retains oral, parenteral feedings (specify calories required for patient) - no vomiting - no significant change in LOC - no undue hyperactivity	• Monitor effects of dietary intake q8h - Monitor I&O q8h: caloric intake, nausea, or vomiting - assess LOC for significant irritability or lethargy q4h • Provide nutritious supplements during and between meals • Provide frequent small snacks, meals • Include patient in dietary management

NURSING DIAGNOSES	OUTCOME CRITERIA	INTERVENTIONS
	• Patient, family discuss typical dietary habits, identify problems, plan for improved methods of nutritional intake	• Assist patient, family to discuss typical dietary habits, to identify problem areas, and to plan for dietary improvements that are feasible to maintain
	• Patient, family identify community resources to foster compliance with required nutritional regimen	• Discuss and provide list of nutrition counseling, teen support groups, free nutrition/feeding centers in community
		RATIONALE: *A high caloric and highly nutritive diet is required to counteract the effects of gastrointestinal side effects associated with drug use.*
3 Sensory/ Perceptual Alterations (visual, auditory, kinesthetic) *r.t. effects of illicit drugs or medications*	• Maintains stable LOC - no hypertension or tachycardia - no significant mood swings - no extreme lethargy - no extreme hyperirritability - no pupillary changes (diplopia)	• Monitor VS q4-6h • Assess LOC baseline; then at 4-8h intervals • Inspect pupils for response to light
	• Experiences no violent outbursts	• Assess mood for depression, hyperactivity, loss of self-control • Administer prescribed medications to produce calming, stabilizing emotional status
	• Experiences no falls	• Monitor LOC q2-4h • Keep padded side rails up or bed in lowest position • Assist to bathroom and other ambulation
		RATIONALE: *Protection from accidental self-harm is essential when the drug produces altered perceptions and balance and when it creates emotional volatility.*

MEDICAL

NURSING DIAGNOSES	OUTCOME CRITERIA	INTERVENTIONS

4 Anxiety
r.t. loss of control, memory loss, fear of withdrawal
	• Participates in discussion of plans for "maintaining" while in hospital
	  - understands primary reason for hospitalization
	  - understands that keeping the chemical dependency in stable state is necessary during hospitalization
		• Monitor for covert illicit drug consumption
		
		• Discuss rationale for treatment of primary diagnosis in conjunction with the secondary problem of chemical dependency
		
		• Reassure that the goal is to avoid "withdrawal" symptoms during hospitalization for a primary acute illness problem
		
		• Discuss need and community resources for follow-up in breaking the chemical dependency

RATIONALE: *A chemical-dependent person who is hospitalized for another primary medical diagnosis needs to understand and to cooperate with dual therapeutic regimens.*

> ***OTHER LESS COMMON NURSING DIAGNOSES:*** Sleep Pattern Disturbance; Fatigue; High Risk for Violence: Self-directed or directed at others; Noncompliance; Powerlessness

ESSENTIAL DISCHARGE CRITERIA

- Is physiologically stable for primary admitting problem
- Is hydrated on oral fluids
- Is alert, oriented

- Affirms need to comply with prescribed dietary plan
- Patient, family affirm need to seek help with chemical dependency, possess list of potential resources

CHRONIC LUNG DISEASE *(Bronchopulmonary Dysplasia)*

NURSING DIAGNOSES	OUTCOME CRITERIA	INTERVENTIONS

1 Impaired Gas Exchange
 	
r.t. ventilation perfusion imbalance
	• Exhibits no s/s of respiratory distress
	  - VS WNL
	  - no pallor or cyanosis
	  - no diaphoresis
	  - minimal retractions
	  - no nasal flaring
	  - no wheezing
	  - no irritability or lethargy
	  - O_2 sats WNL
	  - blood gases WNL
	  - Hb, Hct WNL
		• Assess respiratory parameters q4-8h
		• Monitor blood gases and pulse oximetry
		• Monitor hemoglobin and hematocrit
		• Administer O_2 or mechanical ventilation as ordered
		• Provide adequate nutrition and supplemental iron therapy, if indicated

	• Has decreasing dependence on O_2 and/or mechanical ventilation	• Implement weaning schedule as ordered • Observe tolerance to weaning from respiratory support • Administer steroids as ordered
		RATIONALE: *Alveolar surface area for gas exchange is decreased in chronic lung disease. Careful monitoring of respiratory parameters and early detection of deviations allow for prompt intervention and correction.*

2 Ineffective Airway Clearance
 	
r.t. excessive secretions, increased bronchomotor tone
	• Exhibits no s/s of airway obstruction
	  - no coughing
	  - no wheezing, rales, or rhonchi
	  - no retractions
		• Administer bronchodilators as ordered; note response
		• Suction prn

		RATIONALE: *Prevent further airway obstruction and minimize complications.*

MEDICAL

NURSING DIAGNOSES	OUTCOME CRITERIA	INTERVENTIONS
3 High Risk for Infection *r.t. chronic disease, inadequate acquired immunity*	• Exhibits no s/s of infection - no respiratory distress - no fever - no change in amount, color, odor, or consistency of secretions - no decrease in appetite - no irritability or lethargy	• Minimize exposure of patient to people with respiratory infections • Assess for s/s of infection • Administer routine immunizations; yearly influenza vaccine after 6 months of age
		RATIONALE: *Patients have increased susceptibility to middle ear, sinus, and lung infections; these measures will reduce likelihood of infection.*
4 Fluid Volume Excess *r.t. pulmonary hypertension, CHF*	• Shows no s/s of fluid retention - no respiratory distress - no rales - capillary refill <3 sec - normal peripheral pulses - no tense, bulging fontanel (in infants) - no peripheral edema - no hepatomegaly - no behavioral changes (irritability or lethargy)	• Assess fluid retention parameters q4-8h
	• Has normal BP	• Assess BP daily
	• Gains weight at rate appropriate for age	• Weigh daily on same scale at same time of day • Maintain fluid restrictions • Maintain strict I&O • Administer diuretics as ordered and monitor response
	• Has normal urinary sp. gr.	• Monitor sp. gr. daily
	• Exhibits no metabolic acidosis as shown by blood gases	• Monitor blood gases and serum electrolytes
		RATIONALE: *Early detection and prompt management help prevent fluid overload, electrolyte imbalance, and worsening of respiratory status.*

NURSING DIAGNOSES	OUTCOME CRITERIA	INTERVENTIONS
5 Altered Growth and Development *r.t. increased work of breathing, environmental and stimulation deficiencies*	• Has weight gain of 10-30g (.035-1.05 oz) per day	• Weigh daily on same scale
	• Demonstrates age-appropriate physical growth	• Check height/length weekly • Check head circumference weekly • Plot growth measurements on growth chart as indicated • Consult dietitian about special nutritional needs • Administer high-calorie feedings and nutritional supplements as ordered
	• Demonstrates achievement of appropriate developmental milestones	• Provide age-appropriate toys and activities • Provide tactile, visual, auditory, and social stimuli • Incorporate play into as many aspects of care/interactions as possible
		RATIONALE: *Adequate nutrition is essential to assuring growth and development of critical organ systems. Encouragement of play and activity helps prevent further developmental delays.*
6 High Risk for Activity Intolerance *r.t. respiratory problems/insufficiency*	• Participates fully in ADLs, play, and other therapeutic activities	• Observe for changes in vital signs, color, respiratory effort, behavior, and pulse oximetry readings during activity • Provide frequent rest periods
		RATIONALE: *Adequate rest periods will help prevent hypoxia and progressive respiratory distress.*

MEDICAL

CHRONIC LUNG DISEASE (Bronchopulmonary Dysplasia)

NURSING DIAGNOSES	OUTCOME CRITERIA	INTERVENTIONS
7 High Risk for Altered Parenting *r.t. lack of parental attachment behaviors, growth and development lag, inappropriate response of child to relationships*	• Parents verbalize readiness for child to be discharged	• Encourage parents' involvement in care of child • Prior to discharge, arrange for parents to provide 24-48h of total care • Arrange for multi-disciplinary follow-up as needed (medical specialties, home nursing, respiratory therapy, nutritionist, developmental therapists)

	• Parents demonstrate that they can independently provide all care for child	• Teach parents the essentials of care
		  - pathophysiology and why interventions are important
		  - CPR, emergency plan, home monitoring
		  - medication administration
		  - well-child care
		  - safety needs
		  - respiratory assessment
		  - illness warning signs and appropriate interventions
		  - O_2/mechanical ventilation
		  - special feeding instructions
		  - care of home equipment
		
		• Provide names, phone numbers, and dates for follow-up appointments
		
		• Provide reference list of supplies/medications and instructions for reordering
		
		• Ensure that community supports have been organized (alternative caregivers, support groups, financial support)

		RATIONALE: *Careful instruction and practice are essential so that child will be monitored accurately and appropriate care administered at home. Frequent multi-disciplinary evaluation allows assessment of progress and adjustment of home care plan.*

> **OTHER LESS COMMON NURSING DIAGNOSES:** Dysfunctional Ventilatory Weaning Response; Altered Nutrition: Less than body requirements; Inability to Sustain Spontaneous Ventilation; High Risk for Caregiver Role Strain

ESSENTIAL DISCHARGE CRITERIA

- Exhibits no physiologic compromise with respiratory distress
- Has had no recent increases in respiratory support
- Exhibits sufficient energy for ADLs and play
- Shows no signs of infection or illness

- Parents demonstrate ability to provide all care, list s/s reportable to PCP
- Parents demonstrate understanding of home/community support service

MEDICAL

CLEFT LIP, CLEFT PALATE

NURSING DIAGNOSES	OUTCOME CRITERIA	INTERVENTIONS
1 Altered Nutrition: Less than body requirements *r.t. impaired sucking, swallowing associated with deformity of lip, palate*	• Shows increasing weight, length consistent with normal growth curve	• Weigh daily
	• Takes breast feedings: no excessive stopping, crying, gasping, choking	• For breast feeding, teach mother to manually extend nipple as far as possible
	• Takes bottle feedings: no excessive stopping, crying, gasping, choking	• For bottle feeding, use nipple that allows formula to flow easily; use caution in enlarging hole or fluid will flow too fast
	• Parents demonstrate effective feeding techniques	• Explain how to allow frequent feeding breaks by stopping pressure on bottle, not removing from mouth • Show how to clean mouth thoroughly after feeding; use petroleum jelly for dry lips (unless O_2 in use) • Explain need to position on side or in infant seat (not on abdomen) after feeding • Introduce use of rubber-tipped syringe a few days before surgery to accustom child to postoperative feeding method
		RATIONALE: *Providing feeding breaks reduces infant feeding fatigue and parent frustration. Postfeeding positioning minimizes regurgitation and potential for aspiration.*
2 High Risk for Aspiration *r.t. impaired sucking*	• Parents perform safe and effective positioning methods	• Show how to hold child in sitting position on lap, controlling head with hand and maintaining position at a 45-60° angle • Show how to put child's head slightly forward, chin down • Explain need to burp child before, during, after feeding
		RATIONALE: *Correct anatomical positioning fosters the flow of fluids to the esophagus and minimizes regurgitation.*

NURSING DIAGNOSES	OUTCOME CRITERIA	INTERVENTIONS

3 High Risk for Infection (otitis media, URI)
 	
r.t. compromised primary defenses secondary to malformed palate and eustachian tubes
	• Shows no s/s of infection
	  - has normal body temperature
	  - manifests no excessive mucus, coughing, rubbing ears, irritability, diarrhea
		• Monitor body temperature q4-8h
		• Change position at least q2h •
		• Reinforce good feeding techniques
		• Avoid exposure to URI
		• Teach parents s/s of URI, otitis media
		• Reinforce need for ear exam q3-6 months

		RATIONALE: *Correct feeding techniques prevent aspiration infection. Parents need to be diligent in observing for and obtaining treatment for otitis media. Regular ear and hearing examinations are necessary to prevent uncorrected hearing loss.*
4 High Risk for Altered Parenting *r.t. interrupted bonding secondary to grief, guilt associated with birth of malformed child*	• Parents hold, cuddle child with normal bonding behaviors • Parents express feelings consistent with resolution of loss • Parents participate in infant's care	• Encourage parents to hold, cuddle infant • Encourage parents to express feelings of grief • Explain need to treat infant as normal member of family; role-model acceptance of infant
		RATIONALE: *Encouraging parents to get involved in care and to express their feelings facilitates their grief process, reducing interruptions in bonding process.*
5 Knowledge Deficit *r.t. lack of experience with care requirements*	• Parents express ability to incorporate lifestyle changes into family functioning • Parents express satisfaction with plans for home care • Parents demonstrate correct feeding techniques • Parents list s/s of URI, otitis media	• Assist parents in planning care management at home • Establish partnership with parents in managing feeding techniques • Teach correct feeding techniques • Teach s/s of URI, otitis media

MEDICAL

NURSING DIAGNOSES	OUTCOME CRITERIA	INTERVENTIONS
	• Parents reiterate correct knowledge about surgical repair	• Teach about surgical repair, expected course after surgery
		• Refer to support groups or to social services if parents need financial assistance for care, surgery

RATIONALE: *Demonstrated skills and verbalized confidence increase the likelihood of successful care management at home. Taking a partnership role with parents fosters their self-confidence.*

OTHER LESS COMMON NURSING DIAGNOSES: None

ESSENTIAL DISCHARGE CRITERIA

• Takes feedings without excessive stopping, gasping, choking; gains weight

• Parents demonstrate safe feeding techniques

• Parents list reportable s/s and verbalize confidence in own ability to manage child's care at home

• Parents verbalize plan for follow-up care

CONGESTIVE HEART FAILURE

NURSING DIAGNOSES	OUTCOME CRITERIA	INTERVENTIONS
1 Altered Tissue Perfusion (cardiopulmonary) *r.t. decreased cardiac output secondary to the structural defect or dysfunction causing CHF*	• Displays normalizing stable VS	• Assess VS and cardiac status qh or as indicated • Provide continuous cardiorespiratory monitoring
	• Exhibits warm, dry, pink skin	• Monitor skin color and temperature
	• Displays age-appropriate behavior without SOB	• Assess LOC and age-appropriate behavior

	• Maintains minimum urinary output of 1-3 mL/kg/h	• Monitor urinary output
		• Monitor related lab data
		  - digoxin levels
		  - serum electrolytes
		• Monitor fluid intake
		• Assess response to medications
		  - VS WNL
		  - diuresis
		  - appropriate behavior
		• Administer medications as ordered
		  - inotropics (digoxin)
		  - diuretics (furosemide)
		• Weigh daily, same scale, same time of day

		RATIONALE: *Monitoring changes in the patient's status allows for early identification of problems and subsequent changes in intervention.*
2 Ineffective Breathing Pattern *r.t. pulmonary congestion associated with CHF*	• Maintains normal RR	• Assess RR and effort qh or as indicated
	• Exhibits no increased effort with breathing	• Auscultate breath sounds q2h • Elevate HOB 10-30° • Assess response to medications: diuresis (I&O), decreased edema (usually periorbital in infants), decreased respiratory effort, daily weight
	• Maintains SaO$_2$ WNL	• Monitor pulse oximeter; maintain within perameters

MEDICAL

NURSING DIAGNOSES	OUTCOME CRITERIA	INTERVENTIONS
	• Maintains ABGs WNL	• Monitor ABGs; adminsiter O$_2$ as ordered

	• Rests quietly	• Reduce energy demands
		  - avoid constricting clothing
		  - plan rests between activities
		  - keep crying to a minimum
		  - supplemental O$_2$
		  - feedings

		RATIONALE: *Because tachypnea, a compensatory measure when O$_2$ demands are unmet, is an ineffective breathing pattern for the compromised CHF patient, supplementary O$_2$, medications, and energy conservation measures are required.*
3 Altered Nutrition: Less than body requirements *r.t. increased RR combined with effort of feeding*	• Consumes adequate nutrition to meet growth needs for infants	• For infants: record growth at least weekly on growth charts • For older children: weigh daily
	• Exhibits increase in weight and length	• Obtain and document daily weights
	• Tolerates feedings without fatigue or respiratory distress	• Supplement PO feedings with gavage feedings as ordered • Supplement enteral feedings with parenteral feedings as ordered

	• Parents demonstrate feeding techniques to decrease fatigue
	  - identify signs of distress during feedings/meals and take appropriate action
		• For infants: encourage parents to learn strategies to assist with feeding
		  - hold in semi-sitting position
		  - observe for signs of distress
		  - use small pliable nipple
		  - provide small frequent feedings
		  - increase amount and time between feedings as tolerated
		  - gently burp after feedings
		  - provide supplemetal O$_2$
		• For older children: show parents how to pace spoon feeding to minimize fatigue; offer favorite foods

NURSING DIAGNOSES	OUTCOME CRITERIA	INTERVENTIONS
	• Parents express emotional gratification while feeding infant/child	• If gavage feedings will be required after discharge, teach parents safe gavage feeding techniques
		• Show how to hold and encourage sucking, if tolerated, during feeds
		• Give positive support to parents for taking the time and effort to foster good nutrition
		RATIONALE: *Adequate nutrition is essential for growth and development. Supporting parents with feeding allows family members to experience involvement in meeting child's needs.*
4 **Knowledge Deficit** *r.t. management of an infant with CHF*	• Parents demonstrate active partnership in plan of care	• Develop and implement teaching plan in collaboration with parents
	• Parents identify the cause of CHF, its pathophysiology, and its s/s	• Define CHF and its s/s • Discuss cause of CHF
	• Parents verbalize understanding of therapeutic regimen to increase cardiac output	• Review why child is sick when heart unable to work efficiently
	• Parents discuss plan of care while the child is hospitalized and prepare for discharge • Parents state long-range management goals and prognosis	• Evaluate parents' understanding of long-range management goals; clarify as needed
	• Parents demonstrate a basic understanding of CHF related to the underlying condition	• Outline plan of care to manage CHF while child hospitalized
	• Parents demonstrate understanding of s/s of worsening CHF and when to report to physician	• If child is to be managed at home after initial stabilization, teach - signs of worsening CHF - when to return to physician for further care - strategies for reduction of O_2 consumption during daily care

MEDICAL

NURSING DIAGNOSES	OUTCOME CRITERIA	INTERVENTIONS
	• Parents verbalize understanding of therapeutic regimen to decrease pulmonary congestion	• Teach parents about medications: rationale, dose and time, expected response, potential adverse effects, assessment of pulse before digoxin administration
	• Parents demonstrate strategies to decrease child's O_2 consumption during care activities	• Implement and teach strategies to decrease O_2 consumption - pace care; allow for rest - maintain euthermic environment - treat fever promptly - comfort, alleviate distress or pain when crying - position for comfort and ease of breathing
	• Parents demonstrate proper use of nasal cannula O_2 therapy (if indicated for home care)	• Teach parents home O_2 therapy if planned

RATIONALE: *CHF is a manifestation of ineffective cardiac functioning, frequently caused by a congenital abnormality of the heart in infants. Parents or caregivers need an understanding of the cause and process of CHF to participate in the care, especially if they will care for the child with CHF at home.*

OTHER LESS COMMON NURSING DIAGNOSES: *Impaired Gas Exchange; High Risk for Infection; Altered Growth and Development; Activity Intolerance; High Risk for Aspiration; Ineffective Infant Feeding Pattern; Altered Parenting; Fluid Volume Excess; High Risk for Impaired Skin Integrity; Fatigue; Altered Family Processes; Altered Family Coping*

ESSENTIAL DISCHARGE CRITERIA

- Maintains effective breathing pattern (may require nasal cannula O_2)
- Infant achieves acceptable progressive weight gain
- Parents demonstrate ability to manage cardiac output-related care at home, including appropriate assessments and safe medication administration

- Parents demonstrate ability to provide adequate nourishment and assess effective feeding pattern
- Parents identify indications for seeking medical intervention and for reportable s/s
- Parents possess follow-up appointments

CROHN'S DISEASE

NURSING DIAGNOSES	OUTCOME CRITERIA	INTERVENTIONS
1 Altered Nutrition: Less than body requirements *r.t. the inability to digest food or absorb nutrients due to biological factors*	• Shows weight gain of up to 1 kg (2.2 lb) per week	• Weigh daily
	• Takes normal diet	• Serve meals and snacks around medication schedule when symptoms are controlled • Avoid high-fiber foods and those that aggravate symptoms • Maintain high-protein, high-calorie, low-fat, and low-fiber diet
	• Has normal stools, 1-2/day or as appropriate for age	• Monitor changes in stool consistency
	• Shows normal lab values	• Monitor lab values (CBC, electrolytes, BUN) • Administer meds (sulfasalazine, corticosteroids, antibiotics) as ordered
		RATIONALE: *Correct diet replaces losses and prevents bowel irritation. Body weight and lab values are indicators of nutritional status.*
2 High Risk for Fluid Volume Deficit *r.t. excessive losses from diarrhea or through deviations affecting access to or intake of fluids*	• Maintains balanced I&O	• Monitor, manage strict I&O
	• Maintains stable body weight	• Weigh daily
	• Shows normal urinary sp. gr.	• Monitor urinary sp. gr. q4-8h
	• Achieves normalizing bowel frequency and consistency	• Note amount, frequency, and consistency of all stools
	• Shows no occult blood in secretions, excretions	• Guaiac all stools, emesis, nasogastric drainage
	• Shows normal electrolytes	• Monitor lab values as ordered • Provide oral and parenteral fluids as ordered
		RATIONALE: *Constant monitoring and early detection of fluid loss provide for prompt replacement.*

MEDICAL

NURSING DIAGNOSES	OUTCOME CRITERIA	INTERVENTIONS
3 High Risk for Impaired Skin Integrity *r.t. excretions/secretions, alterations in nutritional state, alterations in metabolic state, medication therapy*	• Displays intact or healing skin	• Check skin daily for tenderness, friction areas, blisters, etc. • Provide warm sitz baths, meticulous perineal care • Consider eggcrate mattress or sheepskin for bed if bedridden • Turn q2-3h if bedridden • Massage skin, bony prominences q2h if bedridden • Avoid any type of donut cushion in bed or chair **RATIONALE:** *Friable skin requires gentle, meticulous cleansing. Prevention of pressure areas reduces skin breakdown.*
4 Powerlessness *r.t. illness-related regimen and unexpected exacerbations*	• Verbalizes and displays control of illness by continuing daily routine and activities as much as possible	• Allow to plan day • Allow time for peer visits • Maintain privacy • Encourage to maintain daily schedule • Encourage to wear own clothes **RATIONALE:** *Focusing on concrete methods to control most elements of his/her own life aids the child to overcome sense of powerlessness.*
5 Anticipatory Grieving *r.t. potential loss or constant changes in future plans due to illness exacerbations*	• Plans at least one activity a week	• Encourage parents and child to plan future activities even when in hospital • Encourage membership in the National Foundation for Ileitis and Colitis, or similar support groups **RATIONALE:** *Planning and implementing specific pleasurable activities reduce sense of loss.*

NURSING DIAGNOSES	OUTCOME CRITERIA	INTERVENTIONS
6 Diversional Activity Deficit *r.t. frequent lengthy treatments and long-term hospitalizations*	• Visits teen lounge in hospital or accepts visitors when hospitalized; talks on phone with friends	• Provide private telephone • Encourage visits to teen lounge • Encourage to make friends on unit **RATIONALE:** *Frequent changes of activity away from hospital routines create diversion from therapeutic regimen.*

7 Altered Family Processes
 	
r.t. child's chronic illness
	• Family develops appropriate coping mechanisms	• Discuss with parents the need to
		  - avoid over-protection
		  - remember the needs of other children in the family
		  - encourage child's independence (in medication, activities, etc.)
		
		RATIONALE: *Coping mechanisms are strengthened by discussing concerns and normalizing family processes.*

8 Anxiety *r.t. change in health status, threat to or change in role functioning, threat to or change in interaction patterns*	• Patient/family verbalize understanding of treatment • Patient/family voice concerns	• Encourage patient and family to discuss Crohn's and how it will affect their life • Involve patient and family in the appropriate support groups **RATIONALE:** *Meeting others with the same problems for discussion and support provides ideas and energy for protecting one's accustomed lifestyle.*
9 Anxiety *r.t. chronic diarrhea, lack of knowledge re: disease process, diagnostic testing, and treatment*	• Uses bedpan or bathroom before soiling occurs; room free of bowel odors	• Provide ready access to bedpan/bathroom • Empty and clean bedpan ASAP after each use • Use room deodorizer • Keep cleansing material available

MEDICAL

NURSING DIAGNOSES	OUTCOME CRITERIA	INTERVENTIONS
	• Verbalizes understanding of the disease process, diagnostic testing, and expected treatment	• Instruct child and family re: normal GI anatomy and physiology • Instruct child and family re: tests and treatments as they are scheduled
		RATIONALE: *Timely bowel control and information can enhance understanding and cooperation and decrease anxiety.*
10 Altered Health Maintenance *r.t. ineffective individual coping, unachieved developmental tasks, denial of illness*	• Verbalizes the "how and why" of Crohn's disease and own medical regimen	• Encourage membership in support groups for patient and family
	• Verbalizes need to keep all doctor appointments	• Encourage patient to take responsibility for medical treatments, dietary regimens, and follow-up appointments
		RATIONALE: *Specific compliance goals and group support foster health maintenance activities.*
11 Altered Sexuality Patterns *r.t. knowledge/skill deficit about alternative responses to health-related transitions or altered body function*	• Verbalizes awareness of need to form relationships with peer group members	• Encourage appropriate sex education • Encourage to wear his/her own clothes even in hospital • Encourage to foster peer relationships with others
		RATIONALE: *Keeping a focus on maintaining normal age-appropriate personal/sexual relationships is important to enhanced self-esteem and to the fostering of normal growth and development.*

> **OTHER LESS COMMON NURSING DIAGNOSES:** *Self-Esteem Disturbance; Knowledge Deficit; Noncompliance; Impaired Social Interaction; Parental Role Conflict*

ESSENTIAL DISCHARGE CRITERIA

- Consumes 90% of normal diet
- Displays normal lab values
- Has normal bowel movements for age
- Maintains satisfactory weight
- Parent/child identify specific support sources, plan for follow-up and s/s reportable to PCP

CROUP

1 Ineffective Airway Clearance

r.t. decreased energy, tracheobronchial infection/secretions

- Demonstrates no s/s of respiratory distress in room air
  - RR 30-40 or baseline for patient
  - no cyanosis, nasal flaring, hoarseness, stridor, retractions, dyspnea
  - ABGs WNL

- Plan activities to allow for rest periods
- Suction only prn
- Push fluids if able to drink; provide IV if not
- Give O$_2$ and humidity as ordered
- Monitor continually for respiratory effort indicating increasing distress
- Provide continuous cardiorespiratory monitoring and pulse oximetry
- Report any increase in RR, hoarseness, cough, retractions, stridor, dyspnea, restlessness, nasal flaring, drooling, or labored and prolonged expirations
- Keep emergency intubation equipment at bedside or in room
- Administer racemic epinephrine treatments if ordered
- Allow child to position self the way he/she is most comfortable

RATIONALE: *Fluids decrease viscosity of tracheobronchial secretions. Constant monitoring of respiratory status facilitates early detection and prompt management of airway obstruction.*

2 Impaired Gas Exchange

r.t. ventilation perfusion imbalance

- Shows no s/s of respiratory distress
  - breath sounds clear and equal bilaterally

- Keep patient as quiet as possible to minimize agitation and decrease the work of breathing
- Auscultate breath sounds q2-4h
- Suction only prn
- Give O$_2$ as ordered
- Monitor continuous pulse oximetry

- Shows normal ABGs

- Monitor ABGs

RATIONALE: *Reducing energy demands helps to reduce respiratory work. O$_2$ and a clear airway aid gas exchange.*

NURSING DIAGNOSES	OUTCOME CRITERIA	INTERVENTIONS
3 Ineffective Breathing Pattern *r.t. decreased energy, fatigue*	• Exhibits normal respiratory pattern and rate	• Assess VS q2-4h • Organize care to allow for as much rest as possible • Allow parents to help in calming patient **RATIONALE:** *Reducing activity and agitation eases work of breathing.*
4 Inability to Sustain Spontaneous Ventilation *r.t. respiratory muscle fatigue*	• Breathes without use of mechanical ventilator	• Observe and monitor ventilatory status qh while on respirator • Maintain artificial airway • Provide continuous cardiorespiratory monitoring • Suction PRN • Insure security of trach/endotracheal tube; re-secure as becomes loosened
	• Shows normal ABGs	• Monitor ABGs • Provide position of comfort; reposition q2-4h as indicated **RATIONALE:** *Artificial ventilation takes over the work of fatigued respiratory muscles.*
5 Impaired Swallowing *r.t. mechanical obstruction, fatigue*	• Consumes and retains 90% of regular diet; swallows secretions	• Allow frequent rest periods during meals, feedings • Assist/select appealing foods • Organize care to allow for maximum rest between feeds **RATIONALE:** *Pacing of feeding combined with frequent rest periods reduce fatigue and enhance swallowing.*

MEDICAL

NURSING DIAGNOSES	OUTCOME CRITERIA	INTERVENTIONS
6 High Risk for Fluid Volume Deficit *r.t. loss of fluid through abnormal routes (indwelling tubes), deviations influencing fluid intake*	• Urinary output is at least 1 mL/kg/h	• Maintain strict I&O • Weigh daily • Provide IVs as ordered; push fluids • Check skin turgor, mucous membranes q4h • Administer analgesic as ordered to decrease any swallowing pain
		RATIONALE: *Monitoring and managing hydration are crucial to recovery. Fever and respiratory effort of croup create high risk for dehydration.*
7 High Risk for Altered Body Temperature *r.t. age, dehydration, inactivity or illness*	• Maintains body temperature at 36.5-38°C (97.7-100.4°F) for 48h	• Monitor temperature q2h • Administer antipyretic as ordered • Monitor I&O • Give tepid sponge bath as ordered for temperature > 40°C (104°F) • Obtain cultures as ordered; monitor results
		RATIONALE: *Antipyretics and tepid sponges cool the body and reduce the risk of dehydration.*
8 Parental Role Conflict *r.t. separation from child due to invasive or restrictive care (intubation)*	• Parents participate in care of the child, both physically and psychologically	• Allow parents to remain with child as much as possible • Allow parents to aid in care e.g., diaper changes, positioning • Follow child's home routine as much as possible (bath in a.m. or p.m., allowed TV shows, story before bedtime)
		RATIONALE: *Parents' active involvement in care and supervision while child is hospitalized puts them in their normal parental roles and reduces effects of restrictive care routines.*

NURSING DIAGNOSES	OUTCOME CRITERIA	INTERVENTIONS
9 Anxiety *r.t. change in health status and threat or change in role functioning*	• Parents/child express concerns	• Encourage family to personalize bedspace
	• Allows staff to comfort him/her	• Discuss parents'/child's fears or concerns
	• Cries less when parents leave	• Allow child to keep his/her favorite toy or stuffed animal in crib
	• Parents participate in child's care and in parental roles	• Allow parents to help set daily routines • Explain all treatments, procedures, and equipment to child and family • Allow parents to remain with child as much as possible • Do not allow parents to assist with painful procedures
		RATIONALE: *When parents are in control of the child's comfort measures, they are less anxious and more able to become competent caregivers in hospital and at home.*

MEDICAL

OTHER LESS COMMON NURSING DIAGNOSES:
High Risk for Injury (internal, biological); Fear (child/parents); Knowledge Deficit

---

ESSENTIAL DISCHARGE CRITERIA

- Shows no s/s respiratory, distress
- Sleeps at least 4 hours at a time
- Takes, retains 90% of diet; demonstrates weight gain

- Parents verbalize knowledge of home care treatment options
- Parents have list of s/s to immediately report or for which to obtain emergency care

CYSTIC FIBROSIS

NURSING DIAGNOSES	OUTCOME CRITERIA	INTERVENTIONS
1 Ineffective Breathing Pattern *r.t. thickened pulmonary secretions, tracheobronchial obstruction*	• Exhibits improving respiratory status - VS return to WNL or baseline - no rales, rhonchi, or wheezes	• Assess VS and auscultate chest q4h
	• Returns to baseline for amount, color of secretions	• Assess characteristics of secretions: quantity, color, consistency, odor
	• Has decreasing hemoptysis	• Estimate amount of blood loss; continue CPT in the presence of mild to moderate hemoptysis
	• Shows no evidence of organisms that are resistant to antibiotics being used	• Monitor sputum culture and sensitivity reports
	• Shows improving skin color • Shows capillary refill < 3 sec	• Observe skin color and capillary refill time
	• Shows improving hydration - normal skin turgor - moist mucous membranes - balanced I&O - normal Hct	• Assess hydration status: skin turgor, mucous membranes, I&O, Hct
		RATIONALE: *Prompt recognition of changes in respiratory status that indicate worsening of patient's condition allows for timely changes in plan of care and prevents the child's condition from deteriorating.*
2 Ineffective Airway Clearance *r.t. bronchial obstruction*	• Shows improving pulmonary function - maintains theophylline levels WNL for weight - improved pulmonary function - normalizing ABGs - mobilizes secretions	• Measure tidal volumes and vital capacity • Administer bronchodilators as ordered; monitor theophylline levels if appropriate • Perform chest physiotherapy or another appropriate airway clearance technique; assist patient with coughing
		RATIONALE: *Managing and monitoring medical pharmacologic interventions and mobilizing secretions through chest physiotherapy improve airway clearance and prevent airway obstruction.*

NURSING DIAGNOSES	OUTCOME CRITERIA	INTERVENTIONS

3 Impaired Gas Exchange
 	
r.t. increased pulmonary secretions
	• Shows decreasing or absence of dyspnea by Days 7-14
	  - no cyanosis
	  - no tachypnea, SOB
	  - alert and oriented
		• Assess level of consciousness, listlessness, and irritability
		• Administer O_2 as ordered via appropriate means
		• Assist child to Fowler's position
		• Stay with child during coughing spells
		• Encourage to ambulate and to turn when in bed

		RATIONALE: *These measures foster gas exchange by improving oxygenation and increasing the body's ability to release CO_2.*
4 Altered Nutrition: Less than body requirements *r.t. impaired pancreatic enzyme release, increased energy requirements from chronic infection and dyspnea*	• Shows decreasing steatorrhea	• Observe stools: amount, color, frequency, consistency
	• Shows normalizing body weight	• Weigh daily
	• Takes, retains 90% or more of meals	• Assess patient's food preferences and plan meals accordingly • Plot on growth curve • Provide high-calorie nutritional supplements bid-qid
	• Number of stools decreases to 2-3/day	• Administer pancreatic enzymes as ordered
	• Shows prealbumin WNL • Has normal mid-arm circumference and triceps skin fold measurements	• Provide a diet that is high in protein, fats, CHO, Na, and calories
	• Shows normal vitamin A and E levels	• Administer vitamins A, D, E, and K
	• Has no vomiting	• Avoid CPT after meals
	• Parents discuss, participate in diet planning	• Teach parents about appropriate diet and nutritional supplements
		RATIONALE: *Improving the patient's nutritional status assists the immune system to fight off infection, promotes normal growth, and increases muscle strength to aid in the work of breathing.*

MEDICAL

NURSING DIAGNOSES	OUTCOME CRITERIA	INTERVENTIONS
5 High Risk for Infection *r.t. decrease in ciliary action and increased pulmonary secretions*	• Maintains normal VS	• Monitor VS q4h, including temperature
	• Shows normal CBC	• Monitor CBC and differential
	• Shows negative cultures	• Obtain sputum for culture and sensitivity
	• Experiences no adverse effects of antibiotics	• Administer antibiotics per orders; monitor for side effects
	• Mobilizes secretions	• Assist with nebulizer treatments and CPT
	• Parents and child verbalize understanding of when to call physician or CF Center: change in sputum characteristics, excessive fatigue, increased cough, increased SOB, fever, chest discomfort, decreased appetite	• Teach child and parents s/s of infection
	• Experiences no nosocomial infection	• Use good handwashing; maintain cleanliness of respiratory equipment
		RATIONALE: *Early detection of infection and prompt management support the ability of the immune system to fight chronic infection and prevent the acquisition of any additional organisms.*
6 Activity Intolerance *r.t. fatigue and dyspnea*	• Tolerates activities; reports, displays no weakness, fatigue upon ADL	• Plan nursing care to allow for rest between activities • Provide progressive increase in activity as tolerated • Problem-solve with patient to develop strategies that conserve energy for performing ADLs
	• Requires decreasing amounts of O_2	• Provide O_2 as ordered prn
	• Sleeps and naps satisfactorily for age	• Change position and provide skin care q2h if on bedrest
		RATIONALE: *Balancing rest and a gradual increase in activity decreases the work of breathing and improves energy levels.*

NURSING DIAGNOSES	OUTCOME CRITERIA	INTERVENTIONS
7 Anxiety (child) *r.t. respiratory distress, hospitalization*	• Exhibits diminishing s/s of anxiety - has relaxed body posture, facial expression - sleeps, naps satisfactorily for age - maintains eye contact	• Assess verbal/nonverbal behavior for s/s of anxiety • Employ other interventions to decrease anxiety: music, art, play, guided imagery, etc. • Encourage parents to stay with child • Provide favorite blanket, toys • Stay with child during dyspneic episodes • Explain all procedures at patient's level of understanding
		RATIONALE: *Monitoring and managing anxiety decrease O$_2$ demand, decrease work of breathing, and make hospitalization less traumatic.*
8 Anticipatory Grieving *r.t. chronic progression of illness, eventual loss of child*	• Parents express feelings, ask questions, participate in discussion of future plans	• Assess family members' psychological status, e.g., fearful, anxious, angry, depressed • Encourage expression of feelings
	• Parents participate in care of child	• Encourage family to play with child and help in child's care
	• Parents participate in support group(s) and/or seek support from other sources	• Assist family to identify, utilize support systems
	• Parents display coping behaviors in dealing with grief	• Observe family for evidence of dysfunctional grieving, such as suicidal ideation, agitation, inability to make decisions; make appropriate referrals for counseling
		RATIONALE: *These observational and support measures assist parents/siblings in their ability to cope and help to minimize the stress of caring for a chronically ill child/sibling.*

MEDICAL

NURSING DIAGNOSES	OUTCOME CRITERIA	INTERVENTIONS
9 Self-Esteem Disturbance *r.t. small size, physical weakness, chronic cough, frequent hospitalizations*	• Asserts self, makes good eye contact, verbalizes or expresses feelings	• Assist child to express self; discuss ways of succeeding; make positive comments about child's strength
	• Is involved in planning own care, makes choices	• Encourage parents to allow child to make independent choices as much as possible
	• Is involved with others with CF	• Introduce child to support network
	• Discusses future: career, schooling, etc.	• Assist child to identify own assets, strengths, and capabilities; assist in planning future • Maintain current peer relationships
		RATIONALE: *Encouraging self-expression, assisting with planning, and introducing sources of support help the child to achieve full potential within the limits of the disease.*

> **OTHER LESS COMMON NURSING DIAGNOSES:** *Diarrhea; Constipation; Decreased Cardiac Output; Self-Care Deficit; Pain (chronic) ; Body Image Disturbance; Fluid Volume Deficit; High Risk for Altered Parenting; Knowledge Deficit*

ESSENTIAL DISCHARGE CRITERIA

• Exhibits effective respiratory effort and improved gas exchange

• Demonstrates effective coughing

• Demonstrates improved nutritional status

• Is afebrile

• Has regular bowel patterns

• Demonstrates the ability to perform ADLs

• Parents verbalize knowledge of home care treatments and list s/s to report to PCP

DIABETIC KETOACIDOSIS

NURSING DIAGNOSES	OUTCOME CRITERIA	INTERVENTIONS
1 Fluid Volume Deficit *r.t. hyperglycemia, osmotic diuresis and/or associated vomiting*	• Displays normalizing, stable VS, BP	• Assess VS, BP q1-4h; place on continuous monitor as ordered; observe for abnormal readings
	• Displays signs of adequate hydration - serum electrolytes WNL - LOC improving, WNL - good skin turgor, moist mucous membranes - urine output WNL - urine negative for ketones - body weight WNL or normalizing	• Monitor serum electrolytes • Assess LOC q2-4h • Inspect skin, mucous membranes q2h x 6 • Maintain strict I&O; administer fluids, electrolytes; monitor effects • Test urine for ketones qh or q void • Weigh daily
		RATIONALE: *Early detection and prompt management of deviation from normal prevent further dehydration, replace losses, and prevent further complications.*
2 High Risk for Injury (internal) *r.t. biochemical effects of hyperglycemia and acidosis*	• Exhibits no hypokalemia, hypophosphatemia, or natremia	• Evaluate electrolytes, serum pH, and orders for fluids, electrolytes, and insulin frequently
	• Achieves balanced I&O	• Monitor I&O
	• Shows normal serum electrolytes	• Administer fluids, electrolytes, and insulin per orders
	• Exhibits acceptable blood sugar level	• Monitor blood sugar, reporting rapid decreases • Physician identifies parameters for acceptable BS fluctuation
	• Shows normal VS, BP	• Monitor VS, BP qh
	• Shows normalizing ketones	• Check urine ketones q1-2h/q void
	• Is alert; exhibits LOC WNL; shows equal, reactive pupils	• Test LOC, pupils, orientation qh; report changes promptly
	• Has stable body weight	• Weigh daily
		RATIONALE: *Insulin corrects acidosis, resolves ketosis, decreases hyperglycemia, and prevents severe complications. Careful monitoring provides data for assessing the effects of insulin dosages.*

MEDICAL

NURSING DIAGNOSES	OUTCOME CRITERIA	INTERVENTIONS
3 High Risk for Injury (internal) *r.t. hyperglycemia secondary to insulin deficit, hypoglycemia*	• Maintains blood sugar within parameters	• Infuse dextrose solution, insulin per orders to maintain blood sugar WNL; notify physician if blood sugar is outside of parameters
	• Shows no s/s of hypoglycemia: sweating, pallor, fatigue, shaking, hunger, mood changes, altered LOC	• Monitor q2h for s/s of hypoglycemic reaction; if taking oral fluids, give fast-acting carbohydrate source PO for low blood sugar • Assess need for additional starch or protein
	• Shows normal VS, BP	• Monitor VS, BP q2h
		RATIONALE: *Frequent monitoring allows early detection and prompt management of hypo/hyperglycemia.*
4 Ineffective Management of Therapeutic Regimen *r.t. complex care requirements* *Refer to "Diabetes Mellitus" care plan*	• Child/parents develop plan for decreasing, preventing the occurrence of further DKA episodes	• Assess level of responsibility for diabetes-related tasks • Reinforce positive, specific plans • Clarify misinformation; give needed information • Help family identify support systems and resources • Provide follow-up (home care, outpatient visits) when indicated
		RATIONALE: *Offering realistic expectations for self-care and providing information will assist family to minimize occurrence of DKA.*
5 Knowledge Deficit *r.t. complex variables in diabetes control, fear of another ketoacidotic episode*	• Parent/child express concerns, discuss disease process: treatment, complications	• Consult diabetic educator, if available • Explain DKA: pathophysiology, treatment, diet, insulin, activity; explain all care, rationale to parents/child
	• Parent/child possess list of s/s of DKA and of s/s of hypoglycemia	• Provide lists of s/s of hyperglycemia, hypoglycemia

NURSING DIAGNOSES	OUTCOME CRITERIA	INTERVENTIONS
		• Provide protocols for hypoglcemic treatment
	• Parent/child select prescribed dietary exchanges from list	• Explain diet requirements • Provide alternative menus from fast foods/popular food items • Consult dietitian
	• Parent/child possess written emergency numbers, follow-up appointments	• Verify possession of emergency phone numbers, follow-up appointments, and knowledge of when to use emergency numbers
	• Parent/child perform safe insulin injection technique	• Demonstrate, explain insulin administration • Obtain return demonstration of insulin administration
	• Parent/child perform blood glucose monitoring and urine ketone testing	• Demonstrate, obtain return demonstration of blood glucose testing and urine ketone testing
	• Parent/child possess "sick day" guidelines (need for increased insulin)	• Demonstrate, obtain return demonstration of blood glucose monitoring

RATIONALE: *Reinforcement and reassurance of parents and child bolster their self-confidence and increase likelihood of successful home care.*

MEDICAL

> ### OTHER LESS COMMON NURSING DIAGNOSES:
> *Altered Tissue Perfusion (cerebral); Family Coping: Potential for growth*

ESSENTIAL DISCHARGE CRITERIA

• Exhibits physiological stability: ketones, serum electrolytes, and blood sugar WNL

• Takes prescribed diet, selects correct foods from list

• Parents/child verbalize correct understanding of DKA: precipitating factors, treatment, complications

• Parents/child demonstrate safe insulin injection technique, urine ketone testing, blood glucose monitoring

• Parents/child express confidence in ability to manage at home or have identified resources for support/assistance

• Parents possess emergency phone numbers, follow-up appointments

DIABETES MELLITUS

NURSING DIAGNOSES	OUTCOME CRITERIA	INTERVENTIONS

1 High Risk for Fluid Volume Deficit
 	
r.t. nausea, vomiting, osmotic diuresis associated with ketoacidosis
	• Manifests adequate hydration
	  - stable weight
	  - good skin turgor
	  - moist mucous membranes
	  - absence of polyphagia, polydypsia, or polyuria
	  - normal LOC
		• Measure urinary output q8h
		• Maintain correct I&O
		• Weigh daily
		• Assess for nausea and vomiting
		• Assess mucous membranes, skin turgor, thirst
		• Offer child appealing forms of fluids within dietary requirements: popsicles, snow cones, jello
		• Offer fluids in colorful containers with interesting straws and use games to encourage fluid intake

	• Manifests no signs of ketoacidosis
	  - no urinary ketones
	  - electrolytes WNL
	  - blood sugar WNL
	  - VS, BP WNL
		• Monitor urine for ketones q void
		• Monitor electrolytes
		• Monitor blood sugar levels before meals and bedtime snack; use blood glucose meter
		• Assess VS and BP q8h
		• Observe for evidence of fruity breath or Kussmaul respirations
		• Administer insulin per orders; observe for effects, side effects
		• Maintain balanced regimen of activity, diet, insulin per orders

		RATIONALE: *Frequent monitoring for s/s of dehydration results in early detection/management. Age-appropriate methods of encouraging fluid intake facilitate child's compliance.*

2 High Risk for Injury
 	
r.t. altered cerebral tissue perfusion (edema) associated with ketoacidosis
	• Exhibits no s/s of cerebral edema
	  - is alert, oriented
	  - has normal pupillary reaction, vision
	  - shows normal gait, demeanor
		• Assess LOC and pupillary reactions q1-4h
		• Assess changes in vision q1-4h
		• Observe for ataxia, irritability, confusion q1-4h

	• Exhibits normal VS, BP	• Monitor VS, BP q1-4h as indicated
		RATIONALE: *Frequent assessment of s/s of cerebral edema results in early detection/management of ketoacidosis and prevents the complication of brain damage.*

NURSING DIAGNOSES	OUTCOME CRITERIA	INTERVENTIONS
3 Knowledge Deficit *r.t. unfamiliarity with diagnosis, complex information*	• Parents/child discuss s/s, causes, treatment of Diabetes Mellitus	• Teach parents about the s/s, treatment, causes of increased blood sugar
	• Parents/child verbalize correct knowledge of - indications for glucagon - actions of insulin - dose adjustments - rules for sick days - waiting times for meals - when to seek help	• Teach parents/child the s/s, treatment, causes of decreased blood sugar • Teach parents/child the s/s, treatment, causes of ketoacidosis • Discuss importance of timely reporting of s/s to PCP
		RATIONALE: *Knowledge of the relationship of blood sugar levels, activity, diet, and insulin is basic to successful management of diabetes. Knowledge of s/s of ketoacidosis is essential to prompt requests for assistance from physician or other care provider.*
4 Knowledge Deficit *r.t. cognitive skills for age levels*	• Parents/child verbalize (and 2- to 5-year-olds demonstrate) basic understanding of disease	• Make referral to child diabetic educator if available; reinforce information • Provide special diabetic teaching coloring book • Make flash cards to reinforce learning content • Teach the "six S's": sleepy, starving, stubborn, shaky, sweaty, spacey • Teach toddler to know s/s and ask for help; use role-playing, coloring books, games • Teach preschooler how to ask for help • Develop situations, questions to test, and reinforce knowledge • Provide praise for correct answers, actions

MEDICAL

NURSING DIAGNOSES	OUTCOME CRITERIA	INTERVENTIONS
	• 6- to 12-year-olds: parents/child verbalize and demonstrate knowledge of disease process	• Make referral to child diabetic educator if possible; reinforce information • Include child in all teaching • Teach age-appropriate content; use appropriate visual aids • Teach the "six S's": sleepy, starving, stubborn, shaky, sweaty, spacey • Provide questions and information applicable to child's own history; refer to diabetic checklist • Develop situations, questions to test and reinforce knowledge (as related to in-depth history) • Provide praise for correct answers, actions
	• 13 years and up: parents/child verbalize and demonstrate knowledge of disease process	• Make referral to diabetic teaching specialist if available; reinforce teaching • Teach age-appropriate content; use appropriate visual aids • Include parents in all teaching • Obtain in-depth history of all daily routines; refer to diabetic checklist • Provide applicable situations and questions to test and reinforce knowledge (as related to in-depth history) • Provide positive feedback for correct knowledge, actions

RATIONALE: *Age-appropriate teaching methods are essential to the parent's/child's ability to successfully manage care at home.*

NURSING DIAGNOSES	OUTCOME CRITERIA	INTERVENTIONS
5 Family Coping: Potential for Growth *r.t. diabetic management adaptation*	• Parents/child verbalize satisfaction with their involvement	• Encourage expression of feelings, questions • Involve parents/child in hospital care regimen • Involve parents/child in evaluation of actual hypo/hyperglycemic episodes

	• Parents/child show agreement, understanding of the care regimen in hospital and at home	• Facilitate home care planning
		  - refer to community support groups
		  - discuss home care situations and help with family anticipatory problem-solving
		  - verify that parents/child have names and numbers of physician, clinic, emergency care facilities
		  - involve home care coordinator in planning

RATIONALE: *Including the parents and child in development of nursing goals and interventions provides them with the necessary decision-making and monitoring skills that are needed at home. Active involvement in the hospital provides the family with a sense of control and comfort that fosters mastery of the learning and coping skills that will be needed for successful care management at home.*

MEDICAL

OTHER LESS COMMON NURSING DIAGNOSES: *Fear (child, family); Altered Nutrition: Greater than body requirements; Noncompliance*

ESSENTIAL DISCHARGE CRITERIA

- Exhibits no extreme fluctuations in blood sugar
- Has balanced I&O
- Parents/child demonstrate correct blood glucose monitoring and urine ketone testing technique
- Parents/child verbalize knowledge of s/s, treatment, causes of hypo/hyperglycemia

- Parents/child identify correct actions for excessive exercise (increased snacks or decreased insulin)
- Parents/child possess identification tag, emergency phone numbers, and follow-up appointments with physician

DIARRHEA, DEHYDRATION

NURSING DIAGNOSES	OUTCOME CRITERIA	INTERVENTIONS
1 Diarrhea *r.t. increased bowel irritability, motility, intestinal inflammation*	• Achieves normal stooling frequency and consistency - formed stool - no pain, cramping associated with stooling - stooling WNL for age	• Identify possible contributing factors: diet, medication, food preparation, and travel • Assess stooling frequency and characteristics - number of stools per day - color, visible blood/mucus - consistency: watery, frothy, thick liquid • Assess degree of pain/cramping • Medicate after each stool or as ordered; collect stool samples as ordered • Provide bowel "rest" or dietary modification as ordered - NPO; IV fluids
		RATIONALE: *Careful monitor of stooling guides nursing and medical management strategies. Medication combined with bowel rest helps to reduce irritations and motility.*
2 Fluid Volume Deficit *r.t. increased abnormal stooling and fluid loss*	• Shows normal hydration - moist mucous membranes - good skin turgor - capillary refill < 3 sec - normal fontanel tension - presence of tears	• Assess for s/s of dehydration q4h
	• Gains or maintains normal weight for age, size	• Evaluate weight (compared with most recent weight prior to onset of diarrhea); weigh daily - 5% wt. loss = mild dehydration - 5-10% = moderate dehydration - 10-15% = severe dehydration
	• Tolerates PO fluid volume • Maintains balanced I&O • Shows urinary sp. gr. WNL • Has urinary output WNL	• Record I&O q8h - time of last voiding: color, volume - weigh diaper q voiding/stooling - monitor urine sp. gr. q8h - monitor urine output q8h

NURSING DIAGNOSES	OUTCOME CRITERIA	INTERVENTIONS

		• Gradually reintroduce nonirritating fluids, food
		  - small volumes of oral electrolyte solution q1-2h
		  - progress to nonirritating liquids and food

	• Is alert, responsive; appropriate orientation for age	• Assess neurological status for orientation, confusion, lethargy, responsiveness
	• Shows normal VS	• Monitor VS including BP
	• Shows normal electrolytes, ABGs, serum glucose	• Monitor lab values; report to physician as indicated
		RATIONALE: *Frequent monitoring and prompt intervention help prevent further fluid imbalance and minimize complications.*

3 High Risk for Impaired Skin Integrity
 	
r.t. repeated perineal contact with acidic stools
	• Displays no evidence of skin breakdown	• Assess for skin irritation
		  - on admission
		  - after each diarrheal stool
		  - during bath
		
		• Teach patient/parents the importance of detecting and preventing skin irritation
		
		• Apply protective barrier as ordered to perineal area; reapply ointment after cleansing
		
		• Wash skin with liquid soap compatible with normal skin pH after each stool; dry thoroughly; allow area to air-dry
		
		• Check q1-2h for incontinence
		
		• Place bedpan or bedside commode within easy access; maintain bed in low position; call light within reach

		RATIONALE: *Techniques for constant, ongoing assessment and consistent preventative measures are required to prevent skin breakdown.*

MEDICAL

NURSING DIAGNOSES	OUTCOME CRITERIA	INTERVENTIONS
4 Knowledge Deficit *r.t. care of child with mild diarrhea and dehydration*	• Parents/child discuss knowledge of dietary control; then ask questions, seek clarification	• Teach parents, child about the other dietary principles for control of diarrhea
	• Parents/child perform and discuss hand washing as a means to control contamination	• Teach family the importance of good hand washing to control possible bacterial contamination and cross-infection
	• Parents discuss reasons for careful hygiene, food storage, regular medical care	• Involve parents in child's care - review food handling - assist to analyze home food preparation, storage - involve parents in feedings - explain need for hygiene
	• Parents verbalize knowledge of follow-up care with physician	• Verify that family has emergency phone numbers, follow-up appointments

RATIONALE: *Knowledgeable, competent parents are likely to comply with care regimen. They are likely to seek medical and other support assistance as needed.*

OTHER LESS COMMON NURSING DIAGNOSES: *Impaired Skin Integrity; High Risk for Altered Body Temperature; Altered Nutrition: Less than body requirements; Pain; Impaired Tissue Integrity; Altered Oral Mucous Membrane*

ESSENTIAL DISCHARGE CRITERIA

• Passes formed stool WNL for age
• Displays no pain, cramping associated with stooling
• Maintains/gains weight

• Has balanced I&O
• Tolerates PO maintenance of fluid volume
• Parents verbalize knowledge and commitment to thorough follow-up

EATING DISORDERS *(Anorexia Nervosa, Bulimia)*

NURSING DIAGNOSES	OUTCOME CRITERIA	INTERVENTIONS
1 Altered Nutrition: Less than body requirements *r.t. anorexia, self-induced vomiting, laxative abuse, distorted perception of body*	• Gains weight of 1 kg (2.2 lb) per week	• Weigh daily in morning before meal, not revealing gains or losses; weigh in gown only; check for concealed weights
	• Shows BUN, serum albumin, Hct, Hb, transferrin, electrolytes normalizing or WNL	• Monitor lab values qd
	• Shows normalizing urine studies for 17 ketosteroids and ketones	• Monitor urinary lab values
	• Has moist mucous membranes	• Assess mucous membranes for dryness q8h
	• Eats 80% or more of each meal	• Increase calories by 200-300/day; not to exceed 3000/day
		• Allow choice of foods (low-calorie foods not allowed)
		• Limit mealtimes to a specific time (40 min)
		• Reduce distractions (conversation, television) during mealtime
		• State time to eat, present food, and state time limit; inform patient that if food is not consumed during a set time, alternate feeding methods will be necessary
		• If food not eaten, start tube feedings
		• Start alternate methods of feeding each time oral food is rejected; be consistent; do not negotiate
		• Withdraw attention at mealtime if child refuses to eat
		• Supervise so as to prevent hoarding of food
		• Avoid giving attention to eating

MEDICAL

NURSING DIAGNOSES	OUTCOME CRITERIA	INTERVENTIONS

	• Agrees to and signs written contract within 1-3 days of admission
	
	• Verbalizes understanding of nutritional requirements
	
	• Takes required number of calories
	
	• Resumes normal eating pattern
		• Provide disciplined environment, behavioral modifications
		  - assign primary caregiver who has associates for all shifts; communicate plans of care to all
		  - make written contract re: child/staff responsibilities for diet/activity/bed rest
		  - expect, anticipate manipulative behaviors regarding feeding

	• Shows decreasing incidence of contract breaks	• Monitor consistency of treatment, compliance
		
		• Provide rewards for weight gain
		  - time with nurse
		  - increased visitor time
		  - social time with other children
		  - access to television, radio, stereo, and/or telephone
		
		• Encourage sense of personal responsibility for success in weight gain

		RATIONALE: *Setting and maintaining strict limits reduce the success of manipulative behavior. Simple, concrete rewards reinforce agreed-upon behaviors.*
2 **High Risk for Fluid Deficit** *r.t. dieting, purging*	• Shows VS WNL	• Monitor VS as required

	• Maintains balanced I&O	• Monitor I&O
		  - observe unobtrusively
		  - keep records at nurse's station

	• Exhibits signs of adequate hydration
	  - moist mucous membranes
	  - good skin turgor
	  - electrolytes WNL
		• Monitor parenteral fluids, electrolytes and TPN
		
		• Stay with patient in bathroom to prevent dumping of fluids

		RATIONALE: *Detection of s/s of dehydration indicates covert purging, dieting.*

NURSING DIAGNOSES	OUTCOME CRITERIA	INTERVENTIONS
3 Body Image Disturbance *r.t. inappropriate fear of obesity, poor self-esteem*	• Shows increased frequency of positive statements about inner strengths and appearance • Begins to verbalize body descriptions as being "thin"	• Provide listening, support - acknowledge child's statements about self-image - redirect to routine topics - make special effort to be a good listener - refer to one team member for discussions of appearance, self-concept - focus on feelings; deal with behaviors
	• Mentions, with increasing frequency, feelings of hunger, thirst, and satiety	• Give praise and support for things well done • Foster successful experiences - begin with easy tasks - focus on positive traits • Encourage patient to express thoughts - have patient draw picture of self - discuss perceptions of self • Encourage good hygiene and grooming for sense of well-being • Respond factually and consistently to questions about diet and nutrition • Encourage and reinforce constructive physical activity • Remind of hunger/satiety before/after meals
	• Participates in physical activities as scheduled	• Incorporate specific type and amount of physical activity as weight gain occurs
	• Experiences prompt detection of food rituals	• Observe for "food rituals," such as eating without lips touching utensils, chewing specific number of times before swallowing
	• Discuss own needs vs. perceived expectations of others	• Increase privileges as child meets expectations
	• Family agrees to be supportive of regimen	• Assess for s/s of dysfunctional family • Refer to social work, pastoral care

RATIONALE: *Reinforcement and support create an environment of powerful positive suggestion which becomes more influential than prior behavioral patterning.*

MEDICAL

115

NURSING DIAGNOSES	OUTCOME CRITERIA	INTERVENTIONS

4 Ineffective Individual Coping
 	
r.t. sense of loss of control, fear of growing up, response to dysfunctional family
	• Displays positive coping behaviors
	  - expresses feelings
	  - identifies stressors; seeks help and support
	  - enacts stress reduction techniques
	  - asserts self with family and significant others
		• Encourage self-expressions, venting of feelings
		
		• Observe, record behaviors that are associated with stress
		
		• Encourage seeking help when stressed
		
		• Assist to identify and then support stress reduction strategies
		
		• Support child's efforts to be assertive when with family
		
		• Encourage significant others to offer consistent support

		RATIONALE: *Stress management and self-assertion help the child to gain positive control. Better control reduces fears and their associated poor coping behaviors.*

5 Ineffective Family Coping: Compromised
 	
r.t. impaired communication patterns, unmet competing needs among family members
	• Responds positively to support of family
	  - identifies needs of other members
	  - describes situations where needs and expectations are unmet (in self and other members)
		• Encourage family and child to express thoughts, feelings, needs
		
		• Assist family to identify areas of disagreement with child
		
		• Reinforce family's listening skills, to hear and acknowledge perceptions of other members
		
		• Emphasize value of taking personal responsibility of using "I" statements
		
		• Redirect family conflict from food to other issues

	• Family and child seek assistance as needed	• Refer to counseling as needed • Provide and discuss list of community resources for continued support
		RATIONALE: *Improved family communication increases each member's understanding of basic issues and fosters family cooperation in seeking help to solve basic issues.*

NURSING DIAGNOSES	OUTCOME CRITERIA	INTERVENTIONS
6 Knowledge Deficit *r.t. lack of information, poor coping skills*	• Expresses, enacts commitment to making lifestyle changes that will maintain normal weight - has fewer contract "breaks" - successfully performs home passes, appointments, positive behaviors - selects own menu that complies with guidelines	• Review, reinforce nutritional requirements, guidelines • Review instructions for managing diet at home - evaluate caloric requirements q2-4 weeks - keep focus on stress management strategies - follow regular exercise regimen
	• Parent/child identify and seek sources of counseling and support - make contact with support persons, groups - identify examples of their own controlling, co-dependent behavior	• Reinforce need for long-term, continued support; involve post-discharge professional to provide continuity • Refer to anorexia group or other source of support • Assist family to initiate, maintain contact with counseling to prevent and minimize co-dependent behaviors within the family group
		RATIONALE: *Securing commitment to long-term follow-up reinforces the family's mutual contract with each other and supports the patient in maintaining her/his newly learned coping skills.*

MEDICAL

OTHER LESS COMMON NURSING DIAGNOSES: *Social Isolation; Noncompliance; Impaired Social Interaction; Altered Family Processes; Altered Sexuality Patterns*

ESSENTIAL DISCHARGE CRITERIA

• Takes 100% of required nutrients orally

• Shows increasing body weight

• Complies with contract with minimal "breaks"

• Parents/child verbalize correct knowledge of dietary, behavioral, counseling regimen; possess follow-up appointments with physician, counselor

• Parents/child have follow-up appointments with support group

• School nurse possesses referral information, list of behaviors to observe as s/s of relapse

EPIGLOTTITIS

NURSING DIAGNOSES	OUTCOME CRITERIA	INTERVENTIONS
1 Ineffective Airway Clearance *r.t. inflammation and obstruction of upper airway (epiglottis)*	• Exhibits normal respiratory status for age - VS WNL - good perfusion - good skin color	• Monitor VS q1-2h and prn while in distress; q4h and prn when not in distress • Assess respiratory status qh when in distress, q2-4h if breathing not labored (include skin color, RR, breath sounds, cough characteristics, respiratory effort, retractions) • Assess respiratory effort with feedings
	• Exhibits good O$_2$ perfusion - O$_2$ sats WNL - sleeps, naps at required, expected intervals for age	• Monitor lab values; report to physician as indicated • Monitor pulse oximeter • Immediately report signs of increasing airway obstruction • Have emergency equipment available (Ambu bag/mask, ET tubes, tracheostomy set-up) • ***Do not*** visualize airway • Administer humidified O$_2$ • Elevate HOB • Maintain quiet, calm environment • Maintain adequate hydration • Provide IV antibiotics as ordered
		RATIONALE: *Visualization of epiglottis may cause spasm and occlusion of airway. Frequent assessment of VS and respiratory status results in prompt detection and management of deviations from acceptable status.*
2 High Risk for Fluid Volume Deficit *r.t. inadequate oral intake, tachypnea, fever*	• Maintains adequate fluid intake - good skin turgor - moist mucous membranes - balanced I&O	• Assess hydration status (skin turgor, mucous membranes) • Record I&O • Encourage oral fluids • Administer IV fluids if patient is unable to tolerate oral fluids • Administer antipyretics for fever control
		RATIONALE: *Children dehydrate quickly; elevated RR and fever can cause large insensible water loss.*

NURSING DIAGNOSES	OUTCOME CRITERIA	INTERVENTIONS

3 Anxiety (high risk for)
 	
r.t. dyspnea, hypoxia, hospitalization
	• Exhibits decreasing anxiety
	  - cooperates in an age-appropriate manner
	  - signs of anxiety/restlessness decrease
		• Do not take child from parent or position of comfort
		• Provide favorite toy or blanket for reassurance
		• Coordinate activities to provide rest
		
		RATIONALE: *The child removed from parent or position of comfort will cry and become more anxious, increasing the work of breathing and the risk of airway obstruction.*

4 Knowledge Deficit *r.t. illness, hospitalization, home care following illness*	• Family demonstrates ability to provide care at home	• Instruct, demonstrate, and obtain return demonstration of how and when to give medications at home **RATIONALE:** *An ineffective home medication routine can exacerbate inflammation or produce an abscess.*

MEDICAL

OTHER LESS COMMON NURSING DIAGNOSES:
High Risk for Infection; Ineffective Breathing Pattern

ESSENTIAL DISCHARGE CRITERIA

- Exhibits no stridor with respirations
- Shows normal temperature, HR, and RR

- Has balanced I&O
- Parents demonstrate ability to provide required care for child

FAILURE TO THRIVE

NURSING DIAGNOSES	OUTCOME CRITERIA	INTERVENTIONS
1 Altered Health Maintenance *r.t. organic/inorganic insufficiencies*	• Has normal or normalizing body weight	• Weigh daily, same scale, same time of day, naked
	• Has normal body temperature, VS	• Monitor VS q4h

	• Shows diminishing s/s of fatigue; no dyspnea, cyanosis with feedings	• Assess for s/s of fatigue, dyspnea (baseline, then qd)
		  - fatigue
		  - listlessness
		  - cyanosis, dyspnea with feeds
		  - abdominal distention
		  - neurologic abnormalities
		  - hyperactivity

	• Takes 90% or more of prescribed nutrients, fluids	• Establish feeding routine
		  - hold child
		  - assign primary nurse as much as possible
		  - establish routine feeding times
		  - provide calming environment for feeds

	• Is alert, oriented; plays with toys, peers	• Provide developmentally appropriate visual/auditory stimulation • Encourage crawling, head-raising activities • Involve parents in care activities
		RATIONALE: *Involving the parents in assessing the child's s/s and then encouraging them to assist with care develop competence in maintaining the child's health in the future.*
2 Altered Nutrition: Less than body requirements *r.t. insufficient intake and/or absorption of nutrients*	• Shows normalizing body weight	• Weigh daily; maintain growth graphic

	• Takes, retains most of prescribed nutrients
	  - diarrhea decreasing
	  - no nausea, vomiting
	  - takes at least 90% of prescribed nutrients, fluids
	  - no muscle flaccidity
		• Monitor for intake, retention of nutrients
		  - assess diarrhea, steatorrhea, emesis q8h
		  - monitor I&O q8h
		  - monitor calorie count q8h
		  - assess muscle tone qd

NURSING DIAGNOSES	OUTCOME CRITERIA	INTERVENTIONS
	• Eats without resistance	• Facilitate intake, retention of nutrients - offer small, frequent feeds - consult dietitian - consult Occupational Therapy
	• Parents participate in feeding	• Include parents in feeding • Give positive feedback for bonding behaviors
		RATIONALE: *Daily monitoring of child's weight and feeding patterns provides data for evaluation of child's status. Involving the parents develops their competence in preventing altered nutrition in the future.*
3 High Risk for Fluid Volume Deficit *r.t. altered fluid intake, diarrhea*	• Maintains balanced I&O	• Maintain strict I&O • Offer favorite fluids frequently • Administer ordered parenterals
	• Shows normal electrolytes • Shows normal urinary sp. gr.	• Monitor electrolytes, urinary sp. gr.
	• Shows decreasing number of loose stools/day	• Assess stools q8h: color, frequency, amount, consistency, guaiac
	• Shows good skin turgor, moist mucous membranes	• Assess skin turgor, mucous membranes q8h
	• Shows normalizing body weight	• Weigh daily or q8h
		RATIONALE: *Careful monitoring of I&O and hydration status fosters prompt, effective hydration management.*

NURSING DIAGNOSES	OUTCOME CRITERIA	INTERVENTIONS

4 High Risk for Impaired Skin Integrity
 	
r.t. malnutrition, dehydration
	• Displays clear, intact skin	• Protect skin
		  - cleanse diaper area frequently; apply protective ointment
		  - bathe daily with mild soap; rinse well
		  - moisturize skin with lubricating cream
		
		RATIONALE: *Meticulous skin care promotes healing of excoriated skin and prevents further skin breakdown.*

5 Altered Parenting *r.t. low self-esteem, inadequate role models combined with fussy, irritable, unhappy child*	• Parents show consistent bonding behaviors • Parents demonstrate consistent eye contact with child	• Assess parents' bonding, attachment behaviors q8h

	• Parents show commitment to learning parenting skills
	  - perform required care
	  - involved in counseling and/or support group
		• Demonstrate feeding, other care techniques
		• Refer to counseling, parenting classes as appropriate
		• Show parents how to provide visual, auditory, tactile stimulation
		• Give positive feedback for positive parenting changes
		
		RATIONALE: *Continued observation of parenting behaviors, support, suggestions, and positive feedback promotes the parents' self-confidence and competence in forming bonding attachments with the child.*

6 Knowledge Deficit *r.t. normal growth and development, child care requirements*	• Parents discuss normal growth and development patterns, identify their child's developmental level	• Explain and discuss patterns of normal growth and development
	• Parents demonstrate skill in assessing child's current and next expected growth and development behaviors/milestones	• Explain how to assess child's growth and development behaviors; describe which behaviors to expect next; provide list of reading material

NURSING DIAGNOSES	OUTCOME CRITERIA	INTERVENTIONS
	• Parents identify community resources: financial, healthcare, support groups; become involved in parenting classes	• Discuss, make list of appropriate community resources: financial, support networks, healthcare
	• Parents verbalize knowledge of follow-up appointments	• Verify parents' knowledge of follow-up appointments

RATIONALE: *The parents may be unaware of or have unrealistic expectations about their child's abilities. The parents' ability to seek and use assistance in the community will aid them in maintaining the child's health in the future.*

OTHER LESS COMMON NURSING DIAGNOSES: Altered Role Performance; Family Coping: Potential for growth; Altered Growth and Development

ESSENTIAL DISCHARGE CRITERIA

- Has stable body weight (at least 80% of ideal for height, frame)
- Takes 90% of nutrients without resistance
- Parents display bonding and attachment behavior with child

- Parents express commitment to treatment plan and list s/s reportable to PCP
- Parents possess follow-up appointments

MEDICAL

FEVER OF UNDETERMINED ORIGIN

NURSING DIAGNOSES	OUTCOME CRITERIA	INTERVENTIONS

1 Hyperthermia
r.t. increased metabolic rate and dehydration associated with undiagnosed illness
	• Shows normalizing body temperature < 38°C (< 100.4°F)	• Monitor VS q4h
		• Keep body temperature < 38°C (< 100.4°F)
		  - dress and cover lightly
		  - provide cooling measures for temperature > 40°C (> 104°F)

	• Develops no complications of fever
	  - seizures
	  - rash, nasal discharge
	  - dry mucous membranes
	  - tachycardia
	  - tachypnea
		• Monitor for s/s of complications q4h
		  - observe LOC, seizures
		  - observe for rash, nasal discharge, changes in apical pulse, RR
		  - assess mucous membranes

		RATIONALE: *Timely management of fever fosters the body's ability to defend and heal itself by reducing the metabolic requirements of high temperature.*
2 High Risk for Fluid Volume Deficit *r.t. increased fluid loss, hypermetabolism*	• Achieves balanced I&O	• Maintain accurate I&O; provide oral, parenteral fluid replacement per orders
	• Displays normal serum electrolytes	• Monitor electrolytes q4h or as ordered
	• Has normal urinary sp. gr.	• Monitor urinary sp. gr. q4h
	• Has stable body weight	• Weigh daily at same time on same scale
	• Displays good skin turgor, moist mucous membranes, normal fontanel tension	• Inspect skin, mucous membranes, fontanels (do not give tepid sponge if s/s of dehydration are present)
		RATIONALE: *Early detection and management of fluid loss prevent dehydration.*

NURSING DIAGNOSES	OUTCOME CRITERIA	INTERVENTIONS

3 Sensory Perceptual Alterations (kinesthetic, visual, auditory) *r.t. altered interferon levels associated with neuroregulation*	• Is alert, oriented; arouses easily	• Monitor LOC q4h for s/s of
		  - disorientation
		  - hallucinations
		  - imbalance
		  - incoordination
		  - listlessness
		  - fatigue

	• Responds appropriately to questions; recognizes parents	• Monitor for behavior changes q4h and prn • Orient child to time, place, person as age-appropriate
	• Parents participate in calming or orienting child	• Explain disorientation to parents; elicit their observations of behavior changes
	• Resumes play activities; rest and sleep qs	• Cluster interventions to allow rest times • Use side rails, soft toys, padding, soft restraints as necessary
		RATIONALE: *Monitoring and managing any disorientation prevents increased energy demands associated with protracted crying and agitation.*
4 Knowledge Deficit *r.t. inexperience with fever management*	• Parents discuss physiology of fevers, treatment rationale, complications; display understanding of diurnal body temperature changes	• Teach, discuss physiology of fevers; explain diurnal variations and definition of "fever"
	• Parents demonstrate skill in taking temperature, giving tepid sponges	• Explain rationale for treatment: antipyretics, tepid sponges, recording status on paper, calling physician if unsatisfactory response to treatment
	• Parents discuss medications: effects, side effects, dosages; state hazards of aspirin for young children	• Explain all ordered medications: effects, side effects, dosage, routes of administration
	• Parents possess emergency numbers, follow-up appointments	• Verify knowledge of follow-up care
		RATIONALE: *Knowledgeable, competent parents are likely to manage home care regimen successfully.*

MEDICAL

> **OTHER LESS COMMON NURSING DIAGNOSES:** *Sleep Pattern Disturbance; Ineffective Thermoregulation; Impaired Gas Exchange; Ineffective Breathing Pattern*

ESSENTIAL DISCHARGE CRITERIA

- Displays moist mucous membranes, good skin turgor, normal fontanel tension
- Parents demonstrate safe skills with temperature-taking, sponge baths, CPR
- Parents list medications: effects, side effects, dosage, and route of administration
- Parents possess emergency numbers, follow-up appointment with physician

NURSING DIAGNOSES	OUTCOME CRITERIA	INTERVENTIONS

1 Fluid Volume Deficit
 	
r.t. rapid fluid loss associated with nausea, vomiting, diarrhea
	• Maintains balanced I&O
	  - normal urinary sp. gr.
	  - normal serum K and NA
		• Monitor, manage strict I&O
		  - check urinary sp. gr. q void, then q8h as it improves
		  - monitor serum electrolytes
		  - expect to give parenteral fluids

	• Maintains stable, normal body weight	• Weigh daily; obtain normal weight from physician's records

	• Exhibits signs of good hydration
	  - good skin turgor
	  - moist mucous membranes
	  - normal fontanel tension
		• Assess hydration q4h: skin turgor, mucous membranes, fontanel

	• Shows daily decrease in diarrhea and emesis, with negative guaiac	• Monitor emesis and stools q4h for frequency, color, and consistency • Accurately measure amounts of excretions • Perform guaiac test on emesis and stools
		RATIONALE: *Children have a higher percentage of body fluid than adults and therefore become dehydrated more easily.*

2 High Risk for Impaired Skin Integrity
 	
r.t. secretions, excretions associated with vomiting, diarrhea
	• Exhibits clear, intact skin	• Protect skin
		  - provide special perineal care: gentle cleansing, protective ointments, heat lamp, medicated creams
		  - avoid use of diaper wipes with alcohol or other irritants; cleanse with soap/water
		  - use cloth diapers prn
		  - provide emesis basin or clean burp pads to prevent skin contact with gastric acids, emesis
		  - massage, lubricate skin prn
		  - use eggcrate mattress if necessary

	• Exhibits intact, moist oral mucosa	• Provide oral care qid: gentle brushing, glycerin swabs, lubricant to lips
		RATIONALE: *Rapid transit time of gastric contents/stools increases the acidic content of the secretions, creating burns to intact skin.*

MEDICAL

NURSING DIAGNOSES	OUTCOME CRITERIA	INTERVENTIONS
3 High Risk for Altered Nutrition: Less than body requirements *r.t. low intake, poor absorption of nutrients*	• Maintains or approaches normal body weight	• Weigh daily

	• Eats at least 80% of prescribed foods, fluids	• Maintain required intake
		  - maintain strict I&O
		  - offer fluids gradually as tolerated, progressing to soft, normal diet
		  - administer parenteral fluids, electrolytes per orders
		  - assess caloric intake: children should take in 1000-2400 calories/day based on age and weight
		  - involve dietitian prn

	• Diarrhea, vomiting is absent or diminishing	• Monitor stools, emesis q8h for frequency, amount, consistency
		RATIONALE: *Rapid transit of stools, vomiting reduce absorption of nutrients. Careful progression of fluids and food maximizes absorption.*
4 Knowledge Deficit *r.t. lack of experience with follow-up care of child*	• Parents reiterate and possess list of s/s of dehydration: dry skin, membranes; vomiting; diarrhea; anorexia	• Describe complications of gastroenteritis; provide list of s/s of dehydration
	• Parents demonstrate feeding, skin care techniques, food handling	• Demonstrate feeding, skin care, food handling
	• Parents can select required nutrients from list	• Review nutrition; explain child's prescribed requirements
	• Parents demonstrate food, formula preparation	• Demonstrate food/formula preparation
	• Parents possess follow-up appointments with nurse, clinic, pediatrician	• Refer to community health nurse prn; verify written follow-up appointments
		RATIONALE: *Although gastroenteritis is common in pediatrics, parents may not understand its causes, the management of this episode, or the management of recurrent episodes.*

OTHER LESS COMMON NURSING DIAGNOSES: *High Risk for Altered Body Temperature*

ESSENTIAL DISCHARGE CRITERIA

- Maintains stable serum Na and K levels

- Has normal or normalizing body weight

- Shows evidence of good hydration: brisk skin elastic recoil, moist mucous membranes, normal fontanel tension

- Passes urine, stools of normal consistency, frequency, amount

- Maintains balanced I&O: takes at least 80% of prescribed foods and fluids orally

- Parents list s/s of dehydration reportable to PCP

MEDICAL

GASTROESOPHAGEAL REFLUX

NURSING DIAGNOSES	OUTCOME CRITERIA	INTERVENTIONS
1 High Risk for Aspiration *r.t. delayed gastric emptying*	• Exhibits normal respiratory status - RR appropriate for age - clear, bilateral breath sounds - O$_2$ saturation WNL - no nasal flaring, tracheal tugging, grunting, cyanosis, diaphoresis, pallor, tachypnea	• Assess patient's respiratory status periodically - assess patient's RR q2-4h and quality of patient's breath sounds - maintain pulse oximeter and notify physician of O$_2$ sats outside of parameters - administer O$_2$ as ordered - assess patient for nasal flaring, tracheal tugging, grunting, cyanosis, diaphoresis, pallor, tachypnea q2-4h - notify physician of respiratory distress
	• Shows no evidence of aspiration	• Position prone or in infant seat with head elevated • Maintain O$_2$ and suction at the bedside • Maintain cardiorespiratory monitor
	• Parents demonstrate knowledge of use of apnea monitor	• Instruct parents in the use of apnea monitor and emergency care in the event that patient would aspirate
		RATIONALE: *Monitoring the patient's respiratory status closely facilitates early intervention to prevent complications. Positioning properly decreases the risk of aspiration by decreasing gastroesophageal reflux.*
2 Potential for Altered Nutrition: Less than body requirements *r.t. frequent vomiting*	• Ingests adequate caloric intake appropriate for age	• Document intake q shift • Document episodes of emesis q shift
	• Gains weight appropriate for age	• Weigh patient daily and record • Place in upright position after feeding (harness, infant seat); prone with mattress elevated • Thicken feedings as ordered; enlarge nipple; notify physician of decreased intake • Notify physician of episodes of emesis • Administer medications as ordered
		RATIONALE: *Monitoring intake is essential to assure normal growth and development. Thickening feedings may decrease the risk of aspiration.*

NURSING DIAGNOSES	OUTCOME CRITERIA	INTERVENTIONS

3 High Risk for Fluid Volume Deficit
 	
r.t. frequent vomiting
	• Maintains adequate hydration
	  - balanced I&O
	  - moist mucous membranes, good skin turgor
	  - urinary output WNL
		• Document PO and IV intake
		• Weigh patient daily and record
		• Assess patient for s/s of dehydration: decreased skin turgor, dry mucous membranes, no tearing, sunken fontanels
		• Monitor urinary output
		• Notify physician for urine output < 1 mL/kg/h

RATIONALE: *Children have a higher percentage of body fluids than adults and therefore become dehydrated more easily.*

OTHER LESS COMMON NURSING DIAGNOSES: *Altered Urinary Elimination; Ineffective Breathing Pattern; Nutrition: Less than body requirements*

MEDICAL

ESSENTIAL DISCHARGE CRITERIA

- Maintains normal respiratory status
- Takes, retains 90% of diet
- Gains weight adequately
- Exhibits signs of adequate hydration

- Parents demonstrate knowledge of monitor use and emergency procedures
- Parents demonstrate effective feeding and positioning techniques and possess follow-up appointments

GUILLAIN-BARRÉ SYNDROME

NURSING DIAGNOSES	OUTCOME CRITERIA	INTERVENTIONS
1 Impaired Gas Exchange *r.t. ineffective breathing secondary to weakness and paralysis of respiratory muscles*	• Maintains an adequate breathing pattern - RR, rhythm, depth WNL - breath sounds clear - skin, mucous membranes, - nail beds normal in color	• Assess rate depth and rhythm of respirations q1-2h • Observe color of skin and mucous membranes q2h • Auscultate breath sounds q2h
	• Exhibits signs of good O_2 perfusion - ABGs WNL - pulse oximetry, O_2 sats WNL - vital capacity WNL for age	• Obtain and monitor ABGs, O_2 sats as ordered • Monitor pulse oximeter qh • Monitor vital capacity q2h • Keep HOB elevated 30° • Encourage coughing/deep breathing q2h while awake • Give supplemental O_2 as ordered • Note any dyspnea, chest pain, or increased restlessness • Notify physician of any changes in respiratory effort or rate, changes in skin color/mucous membranes, or abnormal lab values
		RATIONALE: *Due to progression of disease, the respiratory muscles are affected, which may lead to respiratory failure. Careful monitoring of the patient's respiratory status will help caregivers assess for improved respiration and possibly minimize respiratory complications.*
2 Impaired Mobility *r.t. muscular weakness and paralysis of extremities*	• Participates actively or passively in mobilization one week after admission	• Assess motor strength/functional ability q2-4h; make baseline assessment for comparison
	• Remains free of any complications related to immobility	• Perform passive/(active, if possible) ROM to extremities q2h while awake • Assist with ambulation and transfers from bed to chair • Turn patient q2h • Instruct family members/patient in transfer, turning, and ROM techniques

NURSING DIAGNOSES	OUTCOME CRITERIA	INTERVENTIONS
		• Encourage family participation in care • Provide diversional activities (VCR, video games) • Provide Child Life therapy • Involve physical therapist as ordered; use splints, footboard • Provide safety measures: siderails up, call button within reach
		RATIONALE: *Due to paralysis/weakness of extremities, patients may become immobile. Assisting the patient with maintaining functional abilities in their extremities will help prevent complications such as breakdown, contracture, and loss of joints.*
3 High Risk for Impaired Skin Integrity *r.t. immobility, altered sensation*	• Maintains dry, intact skin; displays healing of any breakdown that occurred prior to admission	• Assess skin condition (color, temperature, turgor and integrity) q4h and prn • Turn q2h; position comfortably • Massage skin/bony prominences q2h to promote circulation • Keep patient clean and dry • Keep linens clean, dry, and wrinkle-free • Utilize devices to minimize pressure on prominent areas
		RATIONALE: *Due to immobility, these patients are at high risk for skin breakdown. Assisting patient and teaching the family and patient techniques to prevent any complications of skin breakdown will help with the recovery phase.*
4 Altered Nutrition: Less than body requirements *r.t. difficulty swallowing/chewing*	• Maintains adequate nutrition - stable body weight - normal lab values - balanced I&O	• Assess patient's ability to chew/swallow on admission and q shift • Weigh daily • Monitor lab values • Maintain strict I&O • Record daily caloric intake

MEDICAL

NURSING DIAGNOSES	OUTCOME CRITERIA	INTERVENTIONS
	• Takes, retains at least 90% of required nutrition	• Provide diet as ordered • Involve patient in dietary choices, noting likes/ dislikes • Encourage self-feeding, if possible, and assist prn • Encourage parental involvement in feedings and making dietary choices • Auscultate bowel sounds q shift; note any abdominal distention • Provide parenteral fluids as ordered • Place NG tube for feedings, as ordered
		RATIONALE: *Close observation and management of nutritional intake can prevent complications such as dehydration or any gastrointestinal problems.*
5 Anxiety *r.t. disease process and sudden change in health status*	• Parent/child voice concerns/ questions related to disease; express confidence in own ability to manage care	• Allow child/family to verbalize feelings and concerns about disease and care being provided • Encourage family's participation in patient's care and decision-making • Deal realistically and honestly with patient and family's anxiety • Offer clear and brief information
		RATIONALE: *Decreasing the patient's and family's level of anxiety by eliciting feelings can enhance their abilities to cooperate with the patient's rehabilitation.*

NURSING DIAGNOSES	OUTCOME CRITERIA	INTERVENTIONS
6 Knowledge Deficit *r.t. complex treatment and prognosis*	• Child/family verbalize knowledge of course of disease	• Allow patient and family to openly discuss feelings, ask questions • Offer pamphlets, fact sheets, or other written material about disease • Determine how much the family knows about the disease • Involve patient and family in the plan of care • Refer family to appropriate support groups
		RATIONALE: *Written information helps to clarify any misconceptions patient and family may have about the diagnosis. Proper information can help family adjust to necessary changes in lifestyle during rehabilitation.*
7 Self-Care Deficit (ADL) *r.t. paralysis of extremities*	• Child/family participate actively or passively in ADLs; ask for assistance as needed by one week post admission	• Encourage patient to perform ADLs independently, if possible • Provide adequate rest periods between activities • Coordinate activities with other members of health team • Provide assistive devices • Encourage family participation • Provide positive feedback for any gain or improvement in patient's care activities • Encourage child and family to verbalize any questions or concerns
		RATIONALE: *Allowing patient/family to participate with ADLs during hospitalization will enhance their competence, helping them to successfully manage the home care and rehabilitation regimen.*

MEDICAL

> **OTHER LESS COMMON NURSING DIAGNOSES:** *Sensory/Perceptual Alterations (specify); Ineffective Individual Coping; Bowel Incontinence; Constipation; Altered Urinary Elimination; High Risk for Activity Intolerance; Impaired Social Interaction*

ESSENTIAL DISCHARGE CRITERIA

- Exhibits spontaneous breathing and normal respiratory function
- Takes, swallows, and retains 90% of required nutrients
- Shows increasing mobility or ability to use assistive devices safely

- Child/family display competence in performing ADLs
- Family identifies community resources that are of specific assistance to their needs
- Parents possess follow-up appointments

HEAD TRAUMA

NURSING DIAGNOSES	OUTCOME CRITERIA	INTERVENTIONS

1 Ineffective Family Coping
 	
r.t. hospitalization, changes in body image, unknown outcomes
	• Displays minimal anxiety and adequate coping skills
	  - parent/child express understanding of illness, hospital routines and care
	  - parent/child discuss concerns or questions
	  - continues with ADL within identified limitations
		• Assess parent/child knowledge of disease process and ability to perform ADL
		• Teach about illness, hospital routines, use of equipment
		• Encourage parent/child to verbalize concerns, questions
		• Encourage to participate in care and decision-making
		• Incorporate home activities with the hospital stay; encourage favorite articles from home (toys, blankets) for sense of security

		RATIONALE: *Knowledge and competence minimize the anxiety of both the child and family in coping with hospitalization and diagnosis.*

2 Altered Tissue Perfusion (cerebral)
 	
r.t. seizure activity, fluid and electrolyte imbalance, hematoma, increased ICP, infection (meningitis/ventriculitis)
	• Maintains LOC appropriate to baseline evaluation
	  - PERL
	  - VS, BP WNL, appropriate for age
	  - respiratory status non-labored and WNL
	  - motor strength within baseline limits
	  - electrolytes WNL
	  - EEG, if ordered, does not indicate status epilepticus
	  - anticonvulsant drug levels within therapeutic range
		• Monitor neuro status, VS q1-4h and prn; report any change in parameters
		• Monitor I&O; maintain fluid restriction, if ordered
		• Monitor electrolytes q4-8h
		• Administer anti-epileptic drugs as ordered; monitor therapeutic results
		• Monitor for seizure activity
		• If status epilepticus is present (seizure activity continuing for 20 min): initiate emergency protocol; anticipate IV anticonvulsant/sedative drug intervention
		• Protect child during seizure activity
		  - position on side
		  - do not attempt to place anything in child's mouth
		  - do not restrain, provide containment
		  - monitor, record process of seizure activity
		  - monitor post-ictal state

		RATIONALE: *Recognize and prevent complications associated with neurologic deterioration.*

MEDICAL

137

NURSING DIAGNOSES	OUTCOME CRITERIA	INTERVENTIONS

3 Altered Nutrition: Less than body requirements
 	
r.t. nausea/vomiting, decreased oral intake
	• Demonstrates adequate nutritional intake
	  - skin turgor elastic and brisk recoil
	  - moist mucous membranes
	  - stable weight (weight WNL for age)
		• Assess child's ability to tolerate oral feedings; if no gag reflex, do not attempt to PO feed
		
		• Provide appropriate diet for age; obtain patient/parent information regarding favorite foods
		
		• Do not administer medications with food or favorite fluids
		
		• Monitor I&O
		
		• Administer parenteral fluids as ordered
		
		• Weigh daily
		
		RATIONALE: *Maintain the high caloric requirements of the pediatric patient.*

4 High Risk for Fluid Deficit
 	
r.t. inability to tolerate fluids and/or fluid restriction
	• Maintains fluid/electrolyte balance
	  - I&O WNL/restriction
	  - electrolyte levels WNL for age
	  - urinary sp. gr. WNL
	  - flat fontanel (infant)
	  - skin turgor elastic/brisk recoil
		• Monitor I&O (urine output 1 to 3 mL per kg body weight per hour)
		
		• Maintain fluid restrictions as ordered
		
		• Weigh daily; monitor and report changes (gain or loss)
		  - 50 g/day (1.75 oz/day) (infant)
		  - 200 g/day (7 oz/day) (child)
		  - 500 g/day (17.5 oz/day) (adolescent)
		
		• Monitor electrolytes q4-8h
		
		• Monitor for dehydration
		  - dry mucous membranes
		  - poor skin turgor
		  - sunken fontanel/eyes
		
		• Monitor urinary sp. gr. as ordered
		
		• Administer parenteral fluids as ordered
		
		RATIONALE: *Fluid and electrolyte imbalance can aggravate, mask neuro signs.*

NURSING DIAGNOSES	OUTCOME CRITERIA	INTERVENTIONS

5 Impaired Skin Integrity
 	
r.t. trauma, surgical wounds
	• Maintains skin integrity
	  - no signs of infection
	  - no CSF leak
		• Assess skin integrity q shift
		• Reposition q2h and prn
		• Maintain clean, dry skin
		• Perform passive ROM q shift and prn
		• Consult OT/PT
		• Notify physician of any bleeding or CSF drainage from wounds, ears, or nose
		• Monitor VS and notify physician of temperature > 38°C (> 100.4°F)

		RATIONALE: *Detect and prevent complications associated with infection and tissue damage.*

6 High Risk for Injury
 	
r.t. limited mobility, decreased muscle tone, paralysis, ataxia, seizure activity, neurologic deficit
	• Is free of injury and maintains optimum mobility within constraints of neurologic deficits
	  - maintains ADL
	  - maintains and improves motor capabilities within identified limitations
		• Assess (upon admission and ongoing) q4-8h
		  - motor activity
		  - muscle strength
		  - muscle tone
		• Monitor skin integrity (clean and dry) q4-8h
		• Maintain extremities in position of function
		• Reposition q2h and prn
		• Consult OT/PT to assist with development of plan of care that maximizes child's potential for achievement
		• Utilize splints and rehabilitative devices as ordered
		• Emphasize to child/parents the importance of maintaining a safe environment (side rails up at all times, supervised play)
		• Provide diversional activity for child within neurologic limitations

	• Parent/child participate in care, identify and perform safety measures	• Encourage active participation in child's ADL; provide stimulation and support to attain difficult tasks

NURSING DIAGNOSES	OUTCOME CRITERIA	INTERVENTIONS
		• Instruct parent/child to maintain a safe environment within the constraints of child's neurologic deficit

RATIONALE: *These measures maximize the child's potential for rehabilitation and prevent further deterioration as a result of neurologic deficit.*

> ***OTHER LESS COMMON NURSING DIAGNOSES:*** *Ineffective Airway Clearance; Altered Urinary Elimination; Knowledge Deficit; Altered Thought Processes; Pain*

ESSENTIAL DISCHARGE CRITERIA

- Displays neurologic status within baseline expectations
- Is free of infection
- Rehabilitation plan is initiated
- Actively participates in ADL within limitations of neurologic deficit

- Parents verbalize plans for home care and follow-up
- Parents list s/s requiring immediate care to PCP

NURSING DIAGNOSES	OUTCOME CRITERIA	INTERVENTIONS

1 Fluid Volume Deficit
 	
r.t. hemorrhage associated with dysfunctional clotting
	• Shows BP and pulse WNL	• Monitor vital signs q2-4h
		  - orthostatic BPs
		  - peripheral pulses
		• Monitor I&O

	• Displays no detectable signs of bleeding	• Check all secretions (urine, stool, sputum) for occult or frank blood

	• Shows clotting factors normalizing	• Assess/monitor pertinent lab value trends
		  - Hb/Hct
		  - coagulation studies (minimum of Factor VIII and PTT levels qd); report any abnormalities
		  - administer blood products as orderd

		RATIONALE: *Monitoring these signs allows for early detection and correction of hemorrhaging.*
2 Pain *r.t. bleeding episodes in joints and muscles*	• Verbalizes/displays effective pain control	• Perform a comprehensive assessment of pain utilizing age-appropriate pediatric pain assessment tools; document q2-4h • Observe for nonverbal cues of discomfort: guarding, moaning, crying, restlessness • Evaluate with child, family, and healthcare team, effectiveness of past pain control measures; integrate previously successful measures into pain management plan

MEDICAL

141

NURSING DIAGNOSES	OUTCOME CRITERIA	INTERVENTIONS

	• Identifies medication or activity that reduces or aggravates discomfort	• Provide pain relief measures; monitor and document effectiveness
		  - administer ordered analgesics on a schedule to prevent breakthrough pain if possible
		  - do not use heat or salicylates for pain relief
		  - reduce or eliminate factors that precipitate or increase perception of pain (i.e., room temperature, lighting, noise, fear)
		  - splint, elevate, and apply cold compresses to affected area
		  - provide comforting, diversional activities (i.e., toys, favorite blanket, stroking, music)
		  - schedule activities to correspond with periods of less pain (after analgesic administration)

		RATIONALE: *Using a consistent assessment tool and a regular schedule of pain management interventions will facilitate increased child comfort.*

3 High Risk for Injury (internal)
 	
r.t. uncontrolled bleeding associated with trauma
	• Sustains no bruising or hemorrhaging from hospital procedures	• Minimize/avoid invasive procedures
		  - SQ, IV, IM injections
		  - rectal temperatures
		  - collect blood via fingerstick, not venapuncture
		• Coordinate essential invasive procedures with administration of cryoprecipitate and Factor VIII concentrates
		• Apply cold compresses to invasive procedure site before and after event
		• Apply fibrin or gelatin foam to bleeding sites
		• Apply pressure to site for minimum of 5 min after event
		• Rotate sites for tourniquet and BP cuffs
		• Use soft toothbrush or toothette for oral care
		• Avoid use of restraints

NURSING DIAGNOSES	OUTCOME CRITERIA	INTERVENTIONS
	• Is free from injury resulting from environmental hazards	• Provide a safe environment - keep bedside rails up - pad bedside rails - have child wear shoes when ambulating - provide soft toys and other diversional activities that do not include sharp implements - use electric razor rather than a straight-edge razor for shaving - use therapeutic mattress to minimize skin trauma - keep environment clear of obstructions
		RATIONALE: *Using safety precautions helps prevent injuries that may result in bleeding episodes.*
4 **Altered Protection** *r.t. chronic hematological abnormality*	• Explains precautions and/or actions needed to protect self/child and prevent bleeding episodes	• Evaluate child's/parents' understanding of the disease process - provide factual information relating to the disease process, its management, and potential outcomes - instruct child/family to wear a medical ID bracelet and notify all healthcare providers of bleeding disorder - identify and plan lifestyle activities to support optimal quality of life, yet prevent injury - instruct family on early signs and symptoms of a bleeding episode • Evaluate amount of stress and coping abilities of child and family - teach child and parents methods for stress management (e.g., relaxation therapy, imagery, counseling, exercise) - encourage spiritual support when desired - identify constructive outlets for emotions/feelings - connect family with appropriate personal and community resources

MEDICAL

NURSING DIAGNOSES	OUTCOME CRITERIA	INTERVENTIONS

RATIONALE: *Children and their families may experience a decreased ability to guard the child from internal or external threats. Assisting the family to adapt to perceived stressors, changes, or threats will help them meet life and disease demands and roles.*

OTHER LESS COMMON NURSING DIAGNOSES: Diversional Activity Deficit; *Impaired Physical Mobility; Impaired Home Maintenance Management*

ESSENTIAL DISCHARGE CRITERIA

- Shows BP and pulse WNL
- Coagulation, Hb, Hct lab values are WNL
- Displays no s/s of bleeding
- Maintains effective pain control

- Parent/child verbalize understanding of disease, treatment, and potential outcomes
- Parent/child identify s/s of early bleeding
- Parent/child identify available personal and community resources

NURSING DIAGNOSES	OUTCOME CRITERIA	INTERVENTIONS
1 Fluid Volume Deficit *r.t. nausea, vomiting, diarrhea, bleeding*	• Maintains balanced I&O	• Monitor, measure I&O • Provide fluids as ordered
	• Has moist mucous membranes; good skin turgor	• Inspect mucous membranes, skin q8h
	• Shows normalizing body weight	• Weigh qd
	• Shows normal Na, K, albumin	• Monitor electrolytes • Administer electrolytes in IV fluids as ordered
	• Has normal abdominal girth	• Measure abdomen at widest part qd, prn (document on Kardex, at bedside exactly where to measure)

	• Shows no evidence of bleeding in stools, urine
	• Displays no bruising, ecchymosis
		• Inspect excretions and skin for s/s of bleeding q8h
		  - guaiac all stools
		  - dip urine for blood

		RATIONALE: *Frequent monitoring results in early detection and prompt management of dehydration and its complications.*
2 Altered Nutrition: Less than body requirements *r.t. anorexia, vomiting, diarrhea, impaired liver function*	• Shows normalizing serum glucose	• Monitor serum glucose
	• Shows normalizing body weight for height, frame	• Weigh daily
	• Achieves balanced I&O	• Monitor I&O; count calories
	• Takes and retains 90% of prescribed amount of calories	• Give medications for nausea, per orders • Assess for s/s of fatigue • Involve dietitian in designing daily nutrition • Provide high-CHO, low-fat diet including vitamins • Obtain input regarding favorite, allowable foods; serve small frequent feedings; largest meal in morning

MEDICAL

NURSING DIAGNOSES	OUTCOME CRITERIA	INTERVENTIONS
		• Involve parents in identifying favorite foods, treats
		• Involve parents in feeding and devising games that encourage nutritional intake
		RATIONALE: *Intense management of nutritional and caloric intake is required to support healing of liver.*
3 High Risk for Injury (internal) *r.t. coagulopathy associated with liver damage*	• Shows no evidence of bleeding - petechiae - prolonged or spontaneous bleeding from venipuncture sites or mucous membranes	• Monitor for signs of coagulopathy
	• Shows no evidence of compromised hemodynamic status - PT, platelet time WNL - VS WNL - no bleeding - Hb, Hct WNL	• Monitor PT, PTT, platelets • Monitor VS q4h • Assess location of blood loss (urine, gastric, stool); report all signs of positive blood results • Monitor Hb/Hct for evidence of blood loss
		RATIONALE: *PT/PTT, platelet count will be abnormal in relation to the extent of liver damage. Assessment enables timely identification of negative trends.*
4 Pain *r.t. abdominal distension, itching, fever*	• Shows stable, normal VS	• Monitor VS q4h
	• Verbalizes, displays reasonable comfort	• Assess level of discomfort q2h • Inspect skin for abrasions (from itching, scratching) q4h • Administer ordered antipyretics, analgesics; assess effects, side effects • Provide tepid sponge baths for fever • Provide age-appropriate distraction, diversion
		RATIONALE: *Monitoring/controlling discomfort reduces metabolic demands, minimizes further catabolism.*

NURSING DIAGNOSES	OUTCOME CRITERIA	INTERVENTIONS
5 High Risk for Impaired Skin Integrity *r.t. pruritus, diarrhea, dehydration, bed rest*	• Has clear, intact skin • Has no redness, breakdown over pressure points • Shows no scratches, abrasions	• Assess skin q8h, prn • Change position q2h • Use eggcrate mattress, soft supportive padding • Give ordered antihistamines, medicated baths • Keep fingernails short, filed
		RATIONALE: *Control of itching and prevention of skin breakdown abrasions minimize metabolic demands associated with discomfort.*
6 Activity Intolerance *r.t. fatigue, imposed bed rest*	• Shows normalizing transaminase levels • Shows stable, normal VS • Increases activity levels without signs of stress, fatigue	• Monitor transaminase levels • Monitor VS q4h • Increase activities as tolerated • Impose bed rest during acute phase • Encourage slowly increasing activities as tolerated • Maintain quiet environment; limit visitors
		RATIONALE: *Normalizing transaminase levels and VS correlates with liver healing, providing a basis for increasing or decreasing activity levels.*
7 Altered Thought Processes *r.t. decreased ammonia excretion, decreased detoxification of nitrogenous wastes*	• Is oriented to time, place, and person • Shows normal ammonia, glucose, BUN	• Monitor for behavioral changes: lethargy, irritability, decreased LOC • Monitor ammonia, blood glucose, and BUN
		RATIONALE: *Hepatic encephalopathy may occur in the early course of the viral illness as a result of an increase in toxins usually metabolized by the liver.*

MEDICAL

NURSING DIAGNOSES	OUTCOME CRITERIA	INTERVENTIONS
8 High Risk for Infection (transmission) *r.t. contagious nature of Virus A & B*	• Remains in isolation until free of active virus	• Utilize universal precautions • Maintain strict isolation procedures per agency protocol, CDC precautions • Enforce strict hand-washing procedures • Maintain strict blood, body fluid procedures • Use disposable utensils
		RATIONALE: *Isolation precautions reduce chance of transmission.*
9 Knowledge Deficit *r.t. inexperience with complex dietary and activity regimen at home*	• Parents/child discuss physiology of disease process, rationale for treatment; demonstrate safe isolation techniques	• Explain hepatitis: pathophysiology, treatment, complications, nutrition, activity, isolation procedures
	• Parents/child select prescribed foods from list	• Involve dietitian in nutrition counseling
	• Parents verbalize commitment to regular follow-up with physician	• Verify parents' commitment to follow-up care • Verify possession of written appointment with physician
		RATIONALE: *Careful follow-up is essential to preventing further liver damage.*

OTHER LESS COMMON NURSING DIAGNOSES: *Diversional Activity Deficit*

ESSENTIAL DISCHARGE CRITERIA

• Exhibits normalizing body weight

• Takes prescribed calories, nutrients

• Parents verbalize knowledge of home care and strategies to minimize transmission

• Parents express confidence in ability to manage care at home

NURSING DIAGNOSES	OUTCOME CRITERIA	INTERVENTIONS
1 High Risk for Infection *r.t. immunodeficiency*	• Is free of s/s of infection - VS WNL - normal appetite - energetic - color appropriate for race	• Assess for s/s of infection - fever - increased pulse and respirations - pallor - lethargy • Monitor VS q4h • Administer antibiotics, antiviral and antifungal medications as ordered • Administer IVIG as ordered
	• Experiences no cough and rhinorrhea	• Use aseptic technique with invasive procedures • Assess for cough, nasal congestion, and adventitious breath sounds q8h • Promote good pulmonary hygiene - inflation of lungs by blowing a balloon or incentive spirometry - turn frequently - gentle oral suction if needed - active play if able
	• Shows WBC with differential WNL	• Monitor CBC with differential qday - watch for neutropenia
	• Displays intact skin without rashes, abrasions	• Assess skin qday for rash, lesions, drainage • Proper hygiene - keep skin clean, dry, and well-lubricated
	• Complies with infection control measures and universal precautions	• Maintain universal precautions; explain precautions to family/visitors • Instruct all visitors to wash hands before and after entering the patient's room • Wash hands before and after caring for the patient to prevent cross-contamination of patients • Wear gloves when contact with blood, body fluids, tissues, non-intact skin, soiled and/or contaminated surfaces is anticipated

MEDICAL

NURSING DIAGNOSES	OUTCOME CRITERIA	INTERVENTIONS
		• Wear gowns when splash with blood or body fluids is anticipated; wear mask and protective eye wear if aerolization or splattering is likely to occur
		• Place used needles and syringes immediately in an impermeable container; do not recap needles
		• Personalize patient contacts by not requiring gloves, gown, or masks when talking with child, taking VS, or in feedings
		RATIONALE: *Early detection and prompt treatment decrease progress of infection. Meticulous compliance with infection control measures protects child from nosocomial and other infections.*
2 High Risk for Infection (transmission) *r.t. contagious nature of virus*	• Remains in isolation until free of active virus	• Utilize universal precautions • Maintain strict isolation procedures per agency protocol, CDC precautions • Enforce strict hand-washing procedures • Maintain strict blood, body fluid procedures • Use disposable utensils
		RATIONALE: *Isolation precautions reduce chance of transmission.*
3 Altered Nutrition: Less than body requirements *r.t. pain, anorexia, diarrhea*	• Maintains or improves body weight	• Weigh daily - use same scale
	• Maintains balanced I&O	• Monitor I&O q8h
	• Has good skin turgor	• Assess skin turgor q8h

NURSING DIAGNOSES	OUTCOME CRITERIA	INTERVENTIONS

| | • Consumes adequate caloric diet | • Encourage intake
  - use creative approaches to enhance intake
  - offer colorful, fun foods
  - encourage family to select/bring in favorite foods
• Provide high-calorie, high-protein diet
• Plan for enteral or parenteral feeding if inadequate intake |

RATIONALE: *Good nutrition enhances growth and development so child will have capacity for normal life.*

---

4 Impaired Gas Exchange

r.t. opportunistic respiratory infections and decreased tidal volume secondary to medication, bacterial pneumonia, anemia

	• Manifests signs of improved/normal gas exchange
	  - has unlabored respirations with normal rate, rhythm, and depth
	  - no nasal flaring, grunting, or retractions
	  - has clear breath sounds with aeration to all lobes
	  - has normal ABGs, O_2 sats
	  - no cyanosis
	  - no tachycardia, tachypnea
	  - no irritability or change in mental status
		• Obtain baseline assessment of respiratory function
		  - assess RR and character, nasal flaring, grunting, or retractions
		  - assess skin color and color of nail beds
		• Monitor ABGs for hypoxemia, O_2 sats for decreased saturation of Hb, and CBC for anemia
		• Assess for signs of impaired gas exchange
		  - cyanosis, tachycardia, tachypnea
		  - anxiety, irritability, change in mental status
		• Position patient for maximum ventilatory efficiency (i.e., high Fowler's position)

	• Demonstrates effective coughing and energy conservation techniques	• Place in cool vapor tent if prescribed • Provide O_2 therapy as prescribed • Increase fluid intake • Assist child to cough effectively using age-appropriate techniques, i.e., chest physiotherapy • Suction airway secretions as needed • Organize activities to allow for rest periods, minimum energy expenditure

NURSING DIAGNOSES	OUTCOME CRITERIA	INTERVENTIONS
		RATIONALE: *Opportunistic infections such as P. carinii, pneumonia, CMV pneumonitis, Mycobacterium Avium Infection, and tuberculosis can create significant lung infections. Positioning, O$_2$ therapy, coughing produce improved ventilation.*

5 Fluid Volume Deficit
 	
r.t. diarrhea secondary to opportunistic bowel infection or medication reaction
	• Displays good hydration
	  - balanced I&O
	  - electrolytes WNL
	  - VS WNL
	  - moist mucous membranes
	  - normal fontanel tension
	  - adequate skin turgor
	  - decreasing number of diarrhea stools
	  - urinary sp. gr. WNL
	  - peripheral pulses palpable
	  - capillary refill < 3 sec
	  - meets minimum hourly urinary output (1-3 mL/kg/h)
		• Administer/monitor IV fluids as prescribed
		• Give fluids as indicated, as tolerated
		• Maintain strict I&O including urine, stool, and emesis
		• Monitor electrolytes; add appropriate electrolytes as prescribed
		• Assess VS, capillary refill time, peripheral pulses, skin turgor, mucous membranes, fontanels q4h
		• Monitor urinary output and sp. gr. q8h or as indicated
		• Encourage PO intake by employing play techniques: cut jello into fun shapes; let child "squirt" juice in mouth with oral syringes

		RATIONALE: *Constant monitoring of hydration produces prompt, effective management. Special attention to games and interesting fluid objects improves oral intake.*

6 Impaired Skin Integrity
 	
r.t. irritant effect of diarrhea stools
	• Has clear, intact skin
	  - exhibits decrease in size and redness of excoriated areas
	  - shows signs of healing in areas of broken skin
		• Change diapers frequently
		• Cleanse buttocks and dry gently each time at diaper change
		• Expose diaper area to air
		• Apply protective ointment

		RATIONALE: *Protection of friable skin requires frequent, gentle cleansing to remove irritating excretions. Drying and ointments protect from further skin damage.*

NURSING DIAGNOSES	OUTCOME CRITERIA	INTERVENTIONS

7 Altered Oral Mucous Membrane
 	
r.t. mucocutaneous lesions secondary to fungal and herpetic infections; mucositis secondary to medication; ineffective oral hygiene
	• Displays intact oral mucosa
	  - absence of thrush
	  - absence of tooth decay
	  - moist mucous membranes
		• Assess mouth for s/s of candidiasis, herpes, hairy leukoplakia, stomatitis, or aphthous ulcers
		• Administer medication as prescribed

	• Parents/child demonstrate effective oral hygiene techniques	• Provide mouth care q2h • Use soft toothbrush or soft mouth swabs to clean teeth, gums, and tongue • Rinse with normal saline q4h and after cleaning mouth • Apply petroleum jelly to lips as needed • Provide soft, bland foods when oral condition is painful; avoid spicy foods • Consider prophylactic medications (ketoconazole, fluconazole) for patients with recurring, persistent thrush • Use oral antiseptic rinses as ordered • Encourage regular dental check-ups
		RATIONALE: *Dry, irritated buccal tissue provides a good medium for bacterial and fungal growth. Frequent cleansing changes the pH of the mouth, thus reducing fungal proliferation.*
8 Hyperthermia *r.t. HIV infection, opportunistic infection, medication*	• Manifests normal body temperature	• Monitor VS, including temperature q2-4h during febrile periods > 38.4°C (101°F) • Assess for acute infection if temperature > 40°C (104°F)

	• Displays optimal comfort during fever
	  - reports/voices reasonable comfort
	  - skin is neither hot nor perspiring
		• Assess breath sounds
		• Assess and document chills, diaphoresis, tachycardia, signs of septic shock
		• Administer antipyretics as ordered
		• Keep child lightly clothed, but do not allow to chill
		• Evaluate need for further cooling measures

MEDICAL

NURSING DIAGNOSES	OUTCOME CRITERIA	INTERVENTIONS
		• Place in lukewarm (not cold) sponge bath if further cooling measure is indicated - cooling blanket as ordered - electric fan - do not let patient chill; do not use alcohol rubs on infants and children • Change linen and bed clothes frequently during periods of diaphoresis
		RATIONALE: *Prompt and continuous management of fever reduces the body's metabolic rate, thus protecting an already vulnerable person from further energy demands.*
9 Altered Growth and Development *r.t. neurologic disease, situational factors*	• Participates in age-related developmental activities - personal/social - language - cognition - motor	• Assess development on a regular basis - developmental milestones - neurologic assessment • Provide stimulation - appropriate toys - play therapy • Encourage parents to interact with child - parents to participate in care/play • Provide opportunity for interaction with others • Consult Child Life specialist
	• Cares for self appropriate to age and condition	• Provide consistent caregiver • Maintain home routine as much as possible • Encourage age-appropriate self-care activities - feeding, bathing, dressing
		RATIONALE: *Sensory deprivation reduces a child's learning, self-testing, and development. Extra stimuli (such as age-appropriate toys, games, videos, and social contacts) minimize sensory deprivation.*

NURSING DIAGNOSES	OUTCOME CRITERIA	INTERVENTIONS
10 Ineffective Family Coping: Compromised *r.t. prolonged disease and progressive disability*	• Parents verbalize fears, feelings, guilt, grief	• Observe parents for expression of grief, fears, guilt - encourage expression of feelings - provide non-threatening environment
	• Parents identify own coping needs - strengths - social support	• Discuss with parents their personal strengths and their coping mechanisms - assist parents to identify social supports
	• Parents involved in decision-making	• Promote decision-making - include parents in care conferences - encourage parents to advocate for child
	• Parents participate in care of child	• Monitor parent-child interactions • Encourage parents to care for child • Foster parenting behaviors - role model parenting skills - encourage verbalizations about parenting - initiate referrals as needed
		RATIONALE: *The stigma of this disease, and potential for others to contract the disease, make for a very challenging family coping.*
11 Knowledge Deficit *r.t. complex home care of child*	• Parent/child explain diagnosis, disease process, and home care needs	• Assess understanding of diagnosis, disease process, and home care - reinforce information
	• Parent/child list medications: purpose, side effects, and dosage	• Explain medications: purpose, side effects, and dosage - provide home schedule
	• Parent/child demonstrate special care needs	• Explain and demonstrate special care needs - involve parents in care
	• Parent/child state s/s of infection - when to seek medical attention	• Review s/s of infection and when to seek medical attention - avoid crowds - avoid contact with ill individuals - hand-washing

MEDICAL

NURSING DIAGNOSES	OUTCOME CRITERIA	INTERVENTIONS
	• Parent/child explain how HIV is transmitted	• Explain HIV transmission - how to prevent transmission • Reinforce normalization of child's lifestyle
	• Parent/child have names and numbers for access to home medical supplies	• Assure parents have access to home medical supplies - provide names and numbers
	• Parent/child identify support persons	• Refer family to support groups as needed

RATIONALE: *Parents who are well-informed will have greater confidence in ability to care for their child.*

OTHER LESS COMMON NURSING DIAGNOSES:
Diarrhea; High Risk for Injury; Anticipatory Grieving; Social Isolation

---

ESSENTIAL DISCHARGE CRITERIA

- Is free of secondary infection
- Consumes adequate caloric intake to maintain stable body weight
- Parents verbalize/demonstrate ability to care for child at home
- Parents list s/s to be reported to PCP

NURSING DIAGNOSES	OUTCOME CRITERIA	INTERVENTIONS
1 High Risk for Injury (internal) *r.t. elevated serum bilirubin levels secondary to RBC breakdown and impaired bilirubin excretion*	• Experiences prompt identification of risk factors (one or more factors present) - prematurity - small for gestational age - Apgar score indicating asphyxia - traumatic delivery - delayed cord clamping - neonatal sepsis - hepatosplenomegaly	• Assess newborn for risk factors on admission
	• Experiences early detection of s/s of hyperbilirubinemia - jaundice - gray stools - dark, concentrated urine - lethargy - poor feeding - sluggish Moro reflex - high-pitched crying - tremors, irritability, seizures	• Assess for s/s of hyperbilirubinemia q1-4h; report s/s
	• Shows stable or decreasing serum bilirubin levels	• Monitor bilirubin levels; report increases of 0.5 mg/dL/h • Provide phototherapy; follow protocols for timing, duration, procedure • Monitor bilirubin level q4-8h while under therapy • Anticipate need for exchange transfusion
	• Shows stable Hb, Hct - Hb 15-24 g % - Hct: 44-64 vol. % (birth); 42-62 vol. % (4-8d)	• Monitor Hb and Hct; report decreases
	• Shows no increase in reticulocytes	• Monitor reticulocytes; report increases

RATIONALE: *Early identification and treatment can minimize side effects of jaundice and severity of disease.*

MEDICAL

157

NURSING DIAGNOSES	OUTCOME CRITERIA	INTERVENTIONS
2 High Risk for Fluid Volume Deficit *r.t. insensible water loss secondary to phototherapy*	• Shows loss of less than 2% of body weight q8h; takes prescribed amount of feedings	• Maintain fluid intake • Continue prescribed feeding schedule • Weigh qd • Monitor I&O • Provide extra oral or IV fluids if excess weight loss, elevated temperature, loose stools, concentrated urine
	• Has urinary output of < 1-3 mL/kg/h - urine color less dark, concentrated - soft, not liquid stools	• Assess output • Monitor color, amount of urine q1-4h • Monitor stools for looseness q1-4h
	• Remains well-hydrated - body temperature WNL - moist mucous membranes - fontanels not depressed	• Assess hydration • Monitor body temperature q2h if on constant monitor, q3-4h with feedings if done manually • Assess mucous membranes, fontanel tension
		RATIONALE: *External heat can cause hyperthermia and dehydration.*
3 High Risk for Impaired Skin Integrity *r.t. phototherapy*	• Has no dermal rash	• Inspect skin q4h; report rash • Use mild soaps for cleaning; avoid abrasive solutions • Turn frequently
	• Shows no irritation of genital skin	• Shield genitals during therapy; keep diaper area clean, dry
		RATIONALE: *An allergic reaction can result from photosynthetic light.*

NURSING DIAGNOSES	OUTCOME CRITERIA	INTERVENTIONS
4 High Risk for Injury (internal) *r.t. conjunctivitis secondary to phototherapy*	• Shows no evidence of conjunctivitis	• Place eye patches on infant during therapy; remove q4h to inspect eyes **RATIONALE:** *Phototherapy places the infant at risk for conjunctivitis. Eye shields provide protection.*
5 High Risk for Injury (internal) *r.t. liver damage secondary to phototherapy*	• Shows no increase in direct bilirubin levels during therapy • Reveals no bronzing of skin, urine	• Monitor direct bilirubin level before each light treatment; report increases • Inspect skin, urine q4h for bronzing; report occurrence **RATIONALE:** *Liver damage can result from the toxic biochemical by-products of bilirubin metabolism and may be evidenced by skin becoming bronze in color.*
6 High Risk for Injury (biochemical, internal) *r.t. exchange transfusion*	• Shows post-transfusion bilirubin levels of no more than half of pre-transfusion level • Maintains normal ranges of BP, HR, temperature during and after procedure • Experiences no aspiration during transfusion • Experiences prompt treatment of cardiac arrest, other critical events	• Monitor pre- and post-transfusion levels of bilirubin, Hb, Hct, other tests as ordered • Monitor bilirubin q4h x 24h post-transfusion, then q8h or per unit standards • Electronically monitor - BP and HR q10min during exchange procedure, q15-30min after procedure for 2h, then routine schedule - temperature using servocontrol or continuous probe • Aspirate stomach before procedure; leave OG/NG open to straight drain • Keep functional resuscitation equipment readily available; administer parenteral fluids per orders

MEDICAL

NURSING DIAGNOSES	OUTCOME CRITERIA	INTERVENTIONS
	• Reveals no evidence of intestinal perforation post-transfusion - bloody stools - abdominal distention - hypotension - cyanosis - vomiting	• Assess for s/s of intestinal perforation per unit standard
		RATIONALE: *Constant monitoring for complications of exchange transfusion fosters prompt detection and management.*
7 High Risk for Altered Parenting *r.t. separation, interrupted bonding*	• Parents display bonding behaviors - feeding - holding - touching - diapering - talking to infant	• Maintain parental contact • Remove from phototherapy for parents' visits as indicated • Encourage parents to feed, hold, diaper infant
	• Parents verbalize feelings, concerns	• Take time to listen to parents' fear, concerns
		RATIONALE: *Normalize bonding by facilitiating close physical contact and parent-infant interactions.*
8 Knowledge Deficit *r.t. lack of experience*	• Parents discuss physiology of condition, treatment rationale	• Provide factual information about physiology of illness - answer questions - clarify misconceptions - provide literature about hyperbilirubinemia
	• Parents ask appropriate questions	• Be alert to inappropriate questions that signal misunderstanding
	• Parents participate in feeding, diapering, holding	• Involve parents in care to maximize skills, confidence with care at home

NURSING DIAGNOSES	OUTCOME CRITERIA	INTERVENTIONS

	• Parents verbalize knowledge of s/s of complications
	  - jaundice in 5-7 days
	  - elevated temperature
	  - lethargy
	  - rigidity of muscles
	  - irritability
	  - high-pitched cry
	  - seizures
	  - poor feeding
		• Discuss s/s of complications; review significance of each symptom

	• Parents identify sources for medical and other follow-up care	• Verify parents' knowledge of follow-up appointments and community resources
		RATIONALE: *Involvement of parents in caregiving and learning about rationale for treatment increases their skill and confidence, and increases likelihood of uneventful recovery at home.*

MEDICAL

OTHER LESS COMMON NURSING DIAGNOSES: Altered Family Processes

---

ESSENTIAL DISCHARGE CRITERIA

- Takes, retains at least 90% of prescribed feedings
- Maintains stable body weight; no less than birth weight
- Parents demonstrate safe, effective infant care
- Parents verbalize plan for infant follow-up

HYPERTENSION

NURSING DIAGNOSES	OUTCOME CRITERIA	INTERVENTIONS
1 High Risk for Injury *r.t. CNS damage associated with uncontrolled hypertension*	• Shows normalizing BP	• Monitor BP q2-4h, prn; select appropriate-size cuff
	• Exhibits no evidence of hypoxia	• Monitor for s/s of hypoxia; administer O_2 prn

	• Manifests stable, improving LOC
	  - is alert, oriented, relaxed
	  - verbalizes, displays absence of headache, dizziness, vision changes
	  - exhibits no head banging or irritability in infants
		• Monitor CNS, LOC; reduce stress
		  - assess LOC, level of irritability q1-2h
		  - deliver ordered medications on time; assess for effects, side effects
		  - elevate HOB
		  - maintain calm, quiet room
		  - reduce excitement, stress
		  - limit caffeine, overeating

		RATIONALE: *Increasing stress raises BP. Increasing BP raises feelings of stress. Preventing and interrupting this hypertensive cycle are important to BP control.*
2 Fluid Volume Excess *r.t. Na retention associated with hypertension*	• Achieves balanced I&O	• Maintain strict I&O
	• Shows serum Na, K WNL	• Monitor electrolytes q8h or as available; monitor K if child on diuretic
	• Manifests no dependent or periorbital edema	• Inspect for dependent or periorbital edema q2-4h
	• Achieves normalizing, stable body weight	• Weigh daily
	• Takes, retains 90% of prescribed diet	• Provide diet as ordered; expect possible Na limitation
		RATIONALE: *Reducing levels of retained fluids aids in decreasing BP. A low-Na diet and diuretics foster the release of excess fluid.*

NURSING DIAGNOSES	OUTCOME CRITERIA	INTERVENTIONS
3 Knowledge Deficit *r.t. complex variables: medications, diet, activity*	• Parents/child express concerns, questions about hypertension	• Encourage expression of concerns, questions; refer to support group
	• Parents/child discuss s/s of increasing BP - headache - dizziness - altered LOC - edema - changes in BP - irritability - head banging in infant	• Explain pathophysiology of hypertension, treatment, complications
	• Parents/child discuss relaxation, activity, diet	• Demonstrate relaxation techniques; explain prescribed diet, activity
	• Parents/child demonstrate accurate BP-taking skills	• Demonstrate BP-taking techniques
	• Parents/child list medications - effects - side effects - toxicity - dosages	• Teach medications: s/s of side effects, toxicity
	• Parents possess phone numbers, required appointments	• Verify knowledge of appointment(s) for follow-up • Encourage faithful, long-term follow-up

RATIONALE: *Family skill and knowledge provide a sense of control and awareness that is essential in promoting understanding and compliance.*

MEDICAL

OTHER LESS COMMON NURSING DIAGNOSES: *Anxiety; Family Coping: Potential for growth*

ESSENTIAL DISCHARGE CRITERIA

- Maintains BP within parameters established by physician

- Parent/child demonstrate BP measurement and documentation

- Parent/child verbalize understanding of:
  - s/s of hypertension and its implications
  - pharmacologic therapies: names of medications, dosages, side effects
  - nonpharmacologic therapies: diet, exercise, weight control

IDIOPATHIC THROMBOCYTOPENIC PURPURA

NURSING DIAGNOSES	OUTCOME CRITERIA	INTERVENTIONS
1 High Risk for Injury *r.t. hemorrhage associated with altered platelet count*	• Shows normal VS, BP	• Monitor VS q2-4h or prn
	• Has platelet count of at least 200,000/mm^3; Hb, Hct WNL	• Monitor platelets, Hb, Hct
	• Exhibits no external bleeding - gums - petechiae - bleeding from puncture sites	• Monitor for s/s of external bleeding q2-4h - inspect skin, gums, puncture sites q2-4h - do not administer IMs or suppositories if platelet count < 30,000/mm^3 - take only axillary or oral temperatures - post venipunctures, apply pressure x 1 min; check q15min x 4
	• Exhibits no s/s of internal bleeding - pallor-cyanosis - clamminess - hematuria - hematemesis - melena - menorrhagia - joint pain	• Monitor for s/s of internal bleeding q2-4h - inspect skin - assess joints for pain - test urine for blood; guaiac all stools
	• Exhibits no s/s of intracranial bleeding - altered LOC - irritability - bradycardia - vomiting - BP increase then sudden decrease	• Monitor LOC and neuro status q2-4h - assess BP
	• Experiences no injuries	• Protect from injury - pad bed rails; provide soft, rounded toys - restrict to safe play activities until platelets increase - use soft toothbrush, soft towels; no dental floss; no straight razors
		RATIONALE: *Frequent monitoring of lab values and observation for manifestations of internal bleeding are crucial to the early detection and prompt management of hemorrhage. Protected play activities and safe utensils and equipment prevent external trauma and hemorrhage.*

MEDICAL

NURSING DIAGNOSES	OUTCOME CRITERIA	INTERVENTIONS
2 High Risk for Injury (internal) *r.t. intestinal, rectal bleeding associated with mechanical injury*	• Has regular, soft, formed bowel movements	• Provide ordered stool softeners; assess effects • Provide high-fluid, high-bulk diet
	• Shows negative Guaiac	• Guaiac all stools
		RATIONALE: *Testing for occult blood in stools helps detect intestinal bleeding. Preventing constipation (hard stools), helps prevent intestinal trauma and bleeding.*
3 High Risk for Infection *r.t. altered immune system*	• Has normal body temperature within 48-72h of antibiotic therapy	• Monitor VS q4h • Administer ordered antibiotics; assess effects
	• Displays no localized erythema	• Inspect skin, puncture sites • Follow agency protocol for prepping venipuncture sites
	• Shows platelets stabilized to at least 200,000/mm^3; WBC WNL	• Monitor platelets, WBC
		RATIONALE: *Frequent monitoring for local and systemic s/s of infection is crucial to obtaining prompt antibiotic therapy.*
4 Anxiety *r.t. hospitalization, fear of prognosis*	• Parents/child verbalize, express fears, concerns; display relaxed body posture, facial expressions	• Encourage expressions of feelings • Be aware that parents of hemorrhage-prone children may be accused of abuse, e.g., suggest that physician provide a letter to Emergency Department when family is out of town
	• Smiles, plays, maintains eye contact	• Treat child normally; discourage rough play
	• Sleeps, naps qs	• Teach bedtime relaxation techniques
	• Parents participate in care	• Involve parents in care of child as much as possible

NURSING DIAGNOSES	OUTCOME CRITERIA	INTERVENTIONS
		RATIONALE: *Children with bleeding and bruising problems often appear to others (including emergency department staff) as though they may be the victims of abuse.*
5 Knowledge Deficit *r.t. fear of recurring hemorrhage*	• Parents verbalize knowledge of disease: etiology, treatment rationale, expected course	• Explain pathophysiology of disease: cause, treatment (including medications), rationale, prognosis
	• Parents discuss s/s of complications: fever, pallor, clamminess, altered LOC, bruising, petechiae, melena, hematemesis, hematuria	• Provide list of s/s of complications to report to physician
	• Parents identify and discuss specific home safety measures	• Review home safety measures; seek parents' input
	• Parents possess emergency phone numbers, follow-up appointments	• Provide emergency phone numbers; review reasons for faithful follow-up care
		RATIONALE: *Knowledgeable, competent parents are likely to safely and effectively manage the child's care at home. They are likely to obtain prompt medical care when indicated.*

MEDICAL

OTHER LESS COMMON NURSING DIAGNOSES: *Fear; Anxiety; Constipation*

ESSENTIAL DISCHARGE CRITERIA

- Shows platelets WNL
- Shows no s/s of bleeding: bruising, petechiae, hematemesis, hematuria, melena

- Parents/child identify specific home safety measures
- Parents possess emergency phone numbers, written follow-up appointments

INFECTIOUS DISORDERS

NURSING DIAGNOSES	OUTCOME CRITERIA	INTERVENTIONS

1 High Risk for Infection
 	
r.t. need for indwelling catheters, dysmaturity, maternal transmission, nosocomial transmission, immune compromise
	• Lab values are WNL
	  - WBC 10,000-20,000
	  - neutrophils 45%
	  - lymphocytes 30%
	  - bands < 10%
	  - band-to-leukocyte ratio < 1:2
		• Monitor lab values; report and discuss variations with physician

	• Cultures are negative	• Administer antibiotics as ordered, according to sensitivities
	• Temperature is WNL	• Provide thermal support as indicated • Monitor axillary temperature q2h or as indicated • Teach caregivers good hand-washing techniques and strategies to minimize cross-contamination
		RATIONALE: *Monitoring prompts early detection and management of infection.*

2 Ineffective Thermo-regulation (neonate)
 	
r.t. infectious process, dysmaturity
	• Axillary temperature is WNL	• Provide thermal support as indicated
		  - servo control
		  - double wall isolette
		  - heat shield
		
		• Assess environmental and axillary temperature q2h or as indicated

		RATIONALE: *Thermal support minimizes system compromise due to temperature instability.*
3 Impaired Tissue Integrity *r.t. fluid support, nutrition, biometric monitoring*	• Displays intact skin and mucous membranes	• Inspect skin q4-8h • Use minimal tape • Use monitoring leads appropriate to size and gestation of child • Remove leads gently

NURSING DIAGNOSES	OUTCOME CRITERIA	INTERVENTIONS
	• IV sites are free of signs of infection	• Inspect IV site(s) qh or as indicated
		• Use aseptic technique when preparing and administering IV fluids and medications
		• Change IV fluids per unit standards; change IV tubing and site per unit standards
		RATIONALE: *Careful technique minimizes the potential for secondary infection.*
4 Pain *r.t. disease process, medication administration, multiple support measures*	• Demonstrates absence of pain - stable VS, neuro status - responds to comfort measures	• Assess child status: VS, neuro
		• Assess stability of HR, respirations, BP
		• Provide comfort measures, e.g., nesting, pacifier, noise reduction
		• Administer pain medication as indicated and ordered
		RATIONALE: *Comfort measures minimize system compromise due to pain stimuli.*
5 High Risk for Infection Transmission *r.t. contagious nature of virus*	• Remains in isolation until free of active virus	• Maintain strict isolation procedures per agency protocol, CDC precautions
		• Enforce strict hand-washing procedures
		• Maintain strict blood, body fluid procedures
		• Use disposable utensils
		RATIONALE: *Isolation precautions reduce chance of transmission.*

MEDICAL

169

NURSING DIAGNOSES	OUTCOME CRITERIA	INTERVENTIONS
6 High Risk for Altered Parenting *r.t. child illness, stress*	• Receives regular visits from parents	• Discuss visiting options with parents/caregivers
	• Receives positive interaction from parents - touching - verbal communication - eye contact	• Teach parents positive interaction strategies relative to child state, status, and ability to receive stimulation
		RATIONALE: *Information, guidance, and support facilitate parenting role.*
7 Knowledge Deficit *r.t. lack of experience with child's condition, course, and management*	• Parents demonstrate knowledge of their child's plan of care	• Discuss disease process with parents/caregivers • Share expectations for anticipated course • Discuss management strategies as they are implemented or questioned by parents
		RATIONALE: *Minimize parent distress by providing information and inclusion in management process.*

> ***OTHER LESS COMMON NURSING DIAGNOSES:*** *Anxiety (parents/caregivers); Fear; Anticipatory Grieving; Powerlessness; Spiritual Distress; Child: Impaired gas exchange; Fluid Volume Deficit; Activity Intolerance; Ineffective Feeding Pattern; Altered Nutrition: Less than body requirements*

ESSENTIAL DISCHARGE CRITERIA

• Is physiologically stable; VS, BP WNL; cultures negative; WBC, platelets, Hb, Hct, clotting factors WNL

• Takes, retains 90% of diet; gains weight

• Parents identify signs of physiologic compromise and demonstrate required care techniques

• Parents identify community health resources, possess written follow-up appointments

INTRACRANIAL PRESSURE, INCREASED

NURSING DIAGNOSES	OUTCOME CRITERIA	INTERVENTIONS

1 High Risk for Injury
 	
r.t. increasing ICP, impaired sensory-motor function, seizures
	• Exhibits no s/s of cerebral injury	• Assess for signs of increasing ICP
		  - altered LOC increases HR, RR, BP (Cushing Striad)
		  - unequal pupil size, sluggish reaction
		  - headache, vomiting
		  - bulging and/or tense fontanels (infants)
		  - increased head circumference
		  - high-pitched cry

	• Maintains adequate cerebral venous outflow
	  - is alert, oriented
		• Elevate HOB 30- 45°
		• Maintain neck in neutral, midline position
		• Minimize coughing, crying, straining (Vasovagal reflex)
		• Decrease environmental stimuli
		  - decrease noise
		  - darken room
		• Maintain normal body temperature
		• Limit and space nursing activities
		• Encourage family members to visit and calm child
		• Place an Ambu bag and O_2 at bedside
		• Keep side rails up when unattended
		• Assist with ADL and ambulating as needed
		• Reorient child as needed
		• Explain to patient/family the need for close supervision

	• Experiences prompt recognition and management of seizures	• Monitor for seizures
		• Pad side rails
		• Administer O_2 as necessary
		• Have suction equipment at bedside if needed
		• Stay with child and remain calm during a seizure
		  - turn head to side
		  - remove harmful objects from area

RATIONALE: *Maintaining positioning and stimuli that foster venous outflow is important to minimizing the effects of increased ICP. Seizures are the most common complication of increased ICP.*

MEDICAL

NURSING DIAGNOSES	OUTCOME CRITERIA	INTERVENTIONS
2 Pain *r.t. headache secondary to increased ICP*	• Is free of pain - VS WNL - limited/no crying, irritability - no complaints of pain	• Assess for presence of headache - voiced complaints - crying, irritability - facial grimacing • Elevate HOB • Dim lights and reduce noise • Place damp cloth on head • Administer analgesics if ordered **RATIONALE:** *Provide comfort measures and adequate pain management.*
3 High Risk for Fluid Volume Deficit *r.t. vomiting, fluid restriction, use of osmotic diuretics*	• Maintains fluid volume WNL - urinary output 1-3 mL/kg/h - urinary sp. gr. WNL for age	• Assess for signs of dehydration - decreased urinary output - increased urinary sp. gr. - dry mucous membranes - poor skin turgor - fever • Maintain accurate I&O • Perform sp. gr. and dipstick on one urine each shift while abnormal • Maintain patent IV • Maintain restricted fluid intake while minimizing dehydration **RATIONALE:** *Consistent monitoring and management of fluid volume reduce risk of dehydration and foster normal fluid balance.*
4 Anxiety *r.t. seriousness of diagnosis, invasive procedures, lack of knowledge*	• Child displays increases psychological and physiologic comfort - vital signs WNL - less irritability, restlessness, and nervousness - improved concentration and sleeping	• Assess family for symptoms of anxiety - physiological: increased HR, RR, BP; diaphoresis, trembling, nausea, vomiting, insomnia, restlessness - emotional: nervousness, helplessness, irritability, crying, withdrawal, anger - cognitive: forgetfulness, inability to concentrate, regression • Offer comfort measures - hold, rock, stroke - offer security object - encourage parents to hold

NURSING DIAGNOSES	OUTCOME CRITERIA	INTERVENTIONS

	• Family displays healthy coping
	  - interest in child, procedures, and tests
	  - interaction with child around ADLs
	  - takes some time away from child to attend own ADLs
		• Assess family's understanding of diagnosis
		  - explain s/s of increased ICP and the need for close monitoring
		  - explain all tests and procedures
		  - clarify and reinforce physician's explanations
		• Encourage family to verbalize feelings and concerns
		• Encourage family to be involved in care of child and to bring familiar objects from home
		• Provide consistent information in a timely manner
		• Encourage parents to care for themselves: rest, nutrition, and time together

RATIONALE: *Patients and families who are encouraged to participate in care and who are well-informed are less anxious.*

MEDICAL

OTHER LESS COMMON NURSING DIAGNOSES:
High Risk for Infection; Ineffective Breathing Pattern; Ineffective Airway Clearance

---

ESSENTIAL DISCHARGE CRITERIA

• Demonstrates improved orientation, LOC

• Seizures are controlled

• Fluid volume is WNL; takes 90% of nutritional requirement

• Achieves pain control

• Parents demonstrate ability able to care for child

• Parents can describe reportable s/s of increased ICP

• Parents possess follow-up appointments

173

JUVENILE RHEUMATOID ARTHRITIS

NURSING DIAGNOSES	OUTCOME CRITERIA	INTERVENTIONS

1 Pain
r.t. joint inflammation
	• Copes with painful joints
	  - exhibits minimal discomfort
	  - able to move with minimal hesitancy
	  - reports pain as tolerable
		• Assess pain level
		  - observe behaviors during play and self-care activities
		  - ask to rate pain on a scale of 1-10 and define acceptance level
		
		• Provide heat to painful joints (tub baths, warm moist pads, soaks) prn
		
		• Avoid overexercising painful, swollen joints
		
		• Administer nonsteroidal anti-inflammatory drugs (NSAIDs) and corticosteroids as ordered

		RATIONALE: *NSAIDs offer analgesic, antipyretic, and anti-inflammatory effects. Heat has a muscle-relaxing effect; heat decreases the viscosity of the synovial fluid and allows improved range of motion in the joint(s).*
2 Impaired Physical Mobility *r.t. joint stiffness, decreased range of motion, discomfort*	• Displays joint mobility, flexibility; is free of deformity	• Assess mobility of joints to establish baseline mobility and to monitor changes
	• Engages in activities appropriate for developmental level, interests, and capabilities	• Implement physical therapy regimen of muscle strengthening and joint mobility exercise, consult OT/PT • Apply heat (warm bath, warm soak, hot pack) before exercising • Administer medication 1h before exercise • Incorporate therapeutic exercises into play, such as: swimming, throwing, riding bicycle, kicking, rolling clay • Encourage maximal independence in activities of daily living/provide devices to facilitate independent functioning
		RATIONALE: *Exercise promotes mobility and maintains function. The application of heat and use of NSAIDs before exercise will decrease discomfort, allowing greater participation.*

NURSING DIAGNOSES	OUTCOME CRITERIA	INTERVENTIONS
3 Altered Growth and Development *r.t. effects of chronic illness and physical disability*	• Performs fine/gross motor skills and demonstrates personal/social behaviors typical for age	• Encourage child and family to emphasize abilities rather than disabilities • Encourage parents to let child assume age-appropriate roles and responsibilities within the family • Encourage participation in peer activities with as few limits as possible • Encourage parents to not be overprotective, but allow child to be exposed to real-life situations and to try new activities; reward independence
		RATIONALE: *Promoting self-worth and independence, setting realistic goals, and establishing open communication allow the child to reach his/her potential in growth and development.*
4 Altered Family Processes *r.t. situational crisis (a child with a chronic illness)*	• Family verbalizes feelings and concerns regarding the disease, needs of the ill child, and the effect on family	• Listen to family members' feelings regarding the child, the illness, and their perception of their ability to cope
	• Family demonstrates attitude of acceptance and confidence in their ability to deal with situation	• Discuss fears with parent/child and siblings • Provide/repeat information regarding the child's illness, limitations, and therapies
	• Family demonstrates knowledge of age-appropriate behaviors and those activities necessary for continued development	• Assist family to achieve a realistic view of the child's capabilities • Reinforce positive aspects of interactions between the child and the other family members • Assist family to gain confidence in their ability to cope with the child, the illness, and the impact on all family members
		RATIONALE: *Children's ability to reach their optimal potential is influenced significantly by their interactions within their family. Family members need support to handle the repeated stresses of a chronic illness and to cope with the situation positively.*

MEDICAL

> **OTHER LESS COMMON NURSING DIAGNOSES:** *Self-Care Deficit (feeding, bathing/hygiene, dressing/grooming, toileting); Activity Intolerance; High Risk for Injury; Fatigue; Self-Esteem Disturbance; High Risk for Ineffective Coping (individual and family); Ineffective Management of Therapeutic Regimen; Knowledge Deficit*

ESSENTIAL DISCHARGE CRITERIA

- Displays minimal or no discomfort when participating in usual daily activities
- Demonstrates age-appropriate behaviors and skills
- Family demonstrates confidence in their ability to care for child; verbalizes knowledge of medications and follow-up appointments

NURSING DIAGNOSES	OUTCOME CRITERIA	INTERVENTIONS

1 High Risk for Infection
 	
r.t. ineffective immune system
	• Exhibits no s/s of infection
	  - temperature < 38°C (< 100.4°F)
	  - negative blood cultures
	  - no signs of infection on physical exam
		• Monitor VS q4h; do not take rectal temps
		
		• Prevent constipation and invasive procedures; no SQ, IM, IV injections
		
		• Obtain blood via fingerstick, not venipuncture
		
		• Double-prep for all required venipunctures
		
		• Inspect skin daily for any areas of breakdown
		
		• Inspect oral cavity for oral candidiasis and breakdowns in the oral mucosal lining
		
		• Monitor WBC and differential daily
		  - pay particular attention to neutrophil count < 500
		
		• Observe for early signs of sepsis
		  - decreasing urine output
		  - significantly high or low temperature
		  - decreasing BP and increasing pulse

	• Parent/child understand the s/s of infection	• Instruct family about s/s of infection and steps to take if infection is suspected • Encourage meticulous oral hygiene
		RATIONALE: *Fever may be the first sign of infection. Intact skin and healthy oral mucosa are the first line of defense against invading organisms. The risk for infection rises as the neutrophil count falls below 500.*
2 Altered Protection *r.t. electrolyte imbalances secondary to tumor lysis*	• Exhibits normal levels of uric acid, K, PO4, Ca; normal BUN, creatinine	• Monitor uric acid, Ca, K, PO4 • Assess for s/s of hypocalcemia • Assess for s/s of hyperkalemia; withhold all K from IV fluids as ordered • Administer allopurinol as ordered - moniter BUN, creatinine • Administer bicarbonate-containing hydration fluids as ordered

MEDICAL

177

NURSING DIAGNOSES	OUTCOME CRITERIA	INTERVENTIONS
	• Maintains balanced electrolytes - balanced I&O - urinary pH > 7.0 - urinary sp. gr. < 1.010	• Maintain strict I&O • Check urinary pH and sp. gr.
		RATIONALE: *Maintaining an alkaline, dilute urine will help the patient excrete uric acid crystals. Allopurinol inhibits production of uric acid.*
3 Activity Intolerance *r.t. impaired O₂ transport secondary to diminished red blood cell count*	• HR WNL for age	• Assess HR and rhythm at least q4h
	• Parent/child understand s/s of anemia and its causes	• Discuss with parent/child s/s of anemia, treatment options • Administer PRBCs as ordered
	• Performs age-appropriate ADL without assistance	• Organize care to allow rest periods
		RATIONALE: *Monitoring and managing O₂ transport fosters activity tolerance.*
4 High Risk for Injury (internal) *r.t. inadequate clotting factors (platelets)*	• Exhibits no evidence of active bleeding from hospital procedures	• Monitor platelet count daily • Inspect stool, urine, gums, emesis, sputum, nasal secretions • Minimize/avoid invasive procedures - SQ, IV, IM injections, punctures - rectal temperatures - coordinate essential invasive procedures with IV of platelets - apply cold compress to site before and after puncture - apply pressure to site for a minimum of 5 min - apply fibrin or gelatin foam to persistently bleeding site - rotate sites for tourniquet and BP cuffs - use soft toothbrush or toothette for oral care - avoid restraints
	• Has bowel movement q1-3 days	• Prevent constipation

NURSING DIAGNOSES	OUTCOME CRITERIA	INTERVENTIONS

	• Is free from injuries resulting from environmental hazards	• Provide a safe environment
		  - have child wear shoes when up ambulating
		  - provide soft toys and other diversional activities that do not include sharp implements
		  - use electric razor rather than razor blade for shaving
		  - keep environment clear of obstructions

	• Parent/child verbalize precautions needed when platelet count is low	• Instruct patient regarding modified age-appropriate activities to minimize risk for trauma
		RATIONALE: *Taking precautions with invasive procedures and providing a safe environment reduce risk of a spontaneous bleed while child is thrombocytopenic (platelets < 30,000).*
5 Anxiety *r.t. unfamiliarity with new diagnosis and treatment plan*	• Parents verbalize concerns about new diagnosis	• Provide parents with lay literature regarding diagnosis and treatment
	• Parents verbalize understanding of treatment plan	• Introduce family to another family whose child has similar diagnosis with similar therapy • Verbally reinforce each day the plan for the next 24-48h

	• Parents verbalize specific reasons to call healthcare team after discharge (especially for temp > 38°C (100.4°F))	• Provide written and verbal discharge instructions
		  - precautions needed at home
		  - reasons to notify healthcare team

		RATIONALE: *A knowledge base regarding diagnosis and treatment will help alleviate the parent's anxiety.*

MEDICAL

OTHER LESS COMMON NURSING DIAGNOSES: *Altered Family Processes;*
Body Image Disturbance; Altered Growth and Development

ESSENTIAL DISCHARGE CRITERIA

- Has temperature < 38°C (100.4°F)
- Has uric acid within normal limits
- Shows no signs of active bleeding
- Shows satisfactory lab values for Hct, neutrophils, platelets
- Parent/child verbalize knowledge of s/s of anemia

- Parent/child verbalize knowledge of s/s of infection
- Parent/child verbalize understanding of necessary precautions while platelet count is low
- Parents verbalize understanding of treatment plan and can identify required sources of support and assistance

MENINGITIS

NURSING DIAGNOSES	OUTCOME CRITERIA	INTERVENTIONS

1 Pain

r.t. meningeal inflammation/irritation, increased ICP

- Exhibits no signs or complaints of pain or meningeal irritation
  - no headache, rigidity, photophobia
  - no excessive irritability
  - normal HR, RR
  - negative Kernig's and Brudzinski's signs

- Assess for signs of meningeal irritation and pain q1-2h

- Shows no s/s of increased ICP
  - exhibits normal VS
  - is consolable
  - displays no irritability
  - makes no complaints of pain
  - exhibits supple neck movements

- Assess for signs of increased ICP q1-2h
  - decreased HR, RR, increased BP
  - altered LOC
  - increased head circumference (infants)
  - full or bulging fontanel (infants)
  - high-pitched cry
  - pupillary changes: unequal, sluggish, dilated
  - headache, vomiting
- Elevate HOB slightly (30-45°)
- Position head midline and stabilize
- Decrease environmental stimuli
  - darken room
  - decrease noise
- Offer comfort measures
  - hold, rock, stroke/massage
  - offer security object
  - encourage parents to hold
- Restrict/limit fluid intake
  - maintain strict I&O
  - use infusion pump to maintain strict IV rate

RATIONALE: *These interventions reduce ICP. When ICP is reduced, pain is lessened.*

2 High Risk for Injury

r.t. seizures secondary to cerebral edema, fever, cortical irritation or damage

- Experiences prompt recognition and management of seizures

- Monitor frequently for seizures

- Sustains no injury during and after a seizure

- Keep side rails up at all times when unsupervised; pad side rails
- Provide only soft toys in bed
- Maintain suction and O_2 at bedside

MEDICAL

NURSING DIAGNOSES	OUTCOME CRITERIA	INTERVENTIONS
		• Stay with child and remain calm during a seizure - turn child to side - remove harmful objects from area - do not try to restrain

RATIONALE: *Seizures are a major complication of meningitis. Should they occur, these protective interventions will help prevent injury.*

NURSING DIAGNOSES	OUTCOME CRITERIA	INTERVENTIONS
3 High Risk for Infection *r.t. exposure to contagious agents, presence of invasive procedures*	• Shows no s/s of infection - temperature WNL - no localized pain, redness, or swelling - WBC count WNL - negative cultures	• Assess for signs of infection - elevated temperature - increased WBC count - positive culture results (blood, urine, CSF) - localized pain, redness, swelling • Maintain a patent IV - restart immediately if infiltrated or inflamed - use aseptic technique • Administer antibiotics in a timely manner • Isolate patient in a private room on mask isolation until 24h of antibiotic therapy is completed.

RATIONALE: *Early recognition and timely antibiotics minimize severity of infection.*

NURSING DIAGNOSES	OUTCOME CRITERIA	INTERVENTIONS
4 Anxiety *r.t. seriousness of diagnosis, invasive procedures, inexperience*	• Child demonstrates increased psychological and physiologic comfort - decreased restlessness, nervousness - limited crying - normal VS - improved sleeping and better concentration	• Assess for symptoms of anxiety - physiologic: increased HR, RR, BP, diaphoresis, trembling, nausea/vomiting, insomnia, restlessness - emotional: nervousness, helplessness, irritability, crying, withdrawal, anger - cognitive: forgetfulness, inability to concentrate, regression • Offer comfort measures - hold, rock, stroke - offer security object - encourage parents to hold

NURSING DIAGNOSES	OUTCOME CRITERIA	INTERVENTIONS

- Parents display healthy coping
  - interest in child, procedures, and tests
  - interaction with child around ADLs
  - take some time away from child to attend own ADLs

- Establish a trusting relationship
  - keep parents informed of child's status
  - involve child in play
  - provide comfort and support during procedures
- Allow parents to remain with child; encourage parents to participate in care
- Provide parents with information regarding diagnosis, tests, and treatment
  - explain and demonstrate any equipment in use
  - answer questions honestly
  - explain all procedures, the reason for them, and their importance
- Provide opportunities for parents to verbalize feelings
- Encourage parents to care for themselves: rest, nutrition, and time together

RATIONALE: *Parents who are well-informed and involved in the care of their child are less likely to be anxious.*

MEDICAL

> **OTHER LESS COMMON NURSING DIAGNOSES:**
> *Fluid Volume Excess; Fluid Volume Deficit; Hyperthermia*

ESSENTIAL DISCHARGE CRITERIA

- Exhibits normal VS, blood count, and cultures
- Maintains manageable pain control

- Parents demonstrate ability to care for child and can identify reportable s/s
- Parents possess follow-up appointments

MENINGOMYELOCELE, REPAIRED *(Older Child)*

NURSING DIAGNOSES	OUTCOME CRITERIA	INTERVENTIONS
1 Altered Tissue Perfusion (cerebral) *r.t. increasing intracranial pressure* *(Refer to "Intracranial Pressure, Increased" care plan)*	• Shows normal, stable VS, BP - pulse WNL for age - respirations regular, unlabored	• Monitor VS, BP q2-4h • Assess respiratory effort
	• Maintains stable neuro status - makes no complaint of headache - is alert, oriented - has no vomiting - PERL	• Assess, manage neuro status
		RATIONALE: *Frequent monitoring of signs of increasing cerebral pressure produces prompt detection and medical management.*
2 High Risk for Infection *r.t. neurogenic bladder*	• Maintains balanced I&O	• Maintain accurate I&O
	• Is afebrile	• Monitor VS q4h
	• Is free of urinary infection - has no urinary frequency, urgency - has clear urine with negative cultures	• Assess for s/s of infection q4h - oliguria - frequency, urgency - cloudy, foul-smelling urine • Report s/s of infection • Provide catheter care
	• Takes at least 90% of required fluids	• Encourage fluids, acidifiers in diet (grape, cranberry, prune juices)
	• Parent/child demonstrate knowledge of catheter care	• Involve child and parents in care; demonstrate and supervise catheter care
		RATIONALE: *Urinary stasis provides a medium for bacterial proliferation, although an indwelling catheter can itself become a potential source of irritation and bacterial transfer.*

NURSING DIAGNOSES	OUTCOME CRITERIA	INTERVENTIONS

3 Bowel Incontinence
 	
r.t. neurogenic bowel
	• Has infrequent involuntary bowel movements; has soft, formed stools	• Assess status of bowel program
		  - make suggestions; provide suppositories, stimulation as ordered
		  - establish regular mealtimes
		  - encourage fluids, roughage, bulk in diet
		  - provide stool softeners

	• Parent/child verbalize, demonstrate knowledge of bowel program	• Review with parents/child the principles of bowel program • Involve parents/child in bowel care
		RATIONALE: *Consistent, vigorous bowel care management helps to prevent hard stools and constipation.*

4 High Risk for Impaired Skin Integrity
 	
r.t. immobility, secretions, excretions
	• Displays clear, intact skin	• Inspect skin under splints, braces, pads q1-2h
		
		• Provide skin care q2h
		  - turn, gradually decreasing turning intervals as child's status requires
		  - use sheepskin, eggcrate, padding in bed
		  - teach to do pressure releases q15-30min when sitting

	• Parent/child discuss and participate in skin care	• Review skin care with parents • Involve parents/child in skin care
		RATIONALE: *Frequent inspection, turning, pressure releases, and protection relieve tissue hypoxia and skin breakdown on pressure points.*

5 Impaired Physical Mobility
 	
r.t. nerve damage associated with meningocele
	• Shows maximum joint mobility
	  - has maximum ROM
	  - has good muscle tone
	  - exhibits steady increase in sitting tolerance
		• Reinforce continuous ROM routine
		  - perform active, passive ROM bid
		  - position in good alignment: use rolls, pillows, pads, splints for support
		  - place in prone position at night and for naps
		  - increase sitting tolerance

MEDICAL

NURSING DIAGNOSES	OUTCOME CRITERIA	INTERVENTIONS
	• Parent/child participate in ROM, alignment	• Demonstrate to parents/child and involve in ROM and alignment techniques
		RATIONALE: *A consistent, well-managed regime of ROM, change of position, and good body alignment prevents joint contractures.*
6 Self-Care Deficit (ADL) *r.t. impaired motor and cognitive function, immobility*	• Maintains prehospitalization bathing, dressing, hygiene, toileting skills	• Monitor, maintain ADL skills - obtain baseline data regarding prehospital ADL: bathing, dressing, toileting - encourage independence - allocate extra time in hospital schedule - teach improved methods of ADL performance; include therapist
	• Parent/child participate in ADL and in fostering independence	• Explain to parents/child the need for independence to the extent possible
		RATIONALE: *Maintaining prehospitalization levels of ADL helps to minimize physical and psychological regression.*
7 Self-Esteem Disturbance *r.t. immobility, deformity, incontinence*	• Participates in own care	• Encourage involvement in own care
	• Verbalizes, displays personal pride in achievements	• Set achievement standards, limits and enforce them
	• Makes positive statements about self; accepts positive reinforcement	• Give positive feedback for positive behaviors; stress strengths, not limitations
	• Asserts self; expresses feelings	• Encourage self-expression, self-assertion
	• Maintains eye contact with family, staff, peers	• Involve family/child in concepts of esteem-building; encourage visits, interactions with siblings, peers

NURSING DIAGNOSES	OUTCOME CRITERIA	INTERVENTIONS
	• Accomplishes (within physical limitations) developmental tasks approximately on time	• Encourage normal developmental activities
		RATIONALE: *The child's active involvement in setting goals promotes maximum self-care independence and enhances self-esteem. Positive feedback, peer interactions, and normalization of lifestyle, to the extent possible, provide the stimulation that fosters normal self-confidence and development.*

8 **Knowledge Deficit** *r.t. supportive home care, prevention of complications*	• Parent/child discuss highest priority problems, solutions	• Assist with problem-solving for home care
		  - discuss previous problems with home care
		  - assist to identify new problems, new solutions

	• Parent/child list reportable s/s: fever; urinary burning, frequency, cloudiness; increasing bowel incontinence; skin breakdown; altered LOC; personality changes	• Describe s/s of complications and why it is important to report to healthcare provider
	• Parent/child demonstrate required care skills	• Teach, demonstrate required care skills
	• Parent/child possess follow-up appointments	• Verify knowledge of follow-up appointments
		RATIONALE: *Competent parents are likely to provide the child with safe, uneventful rehabilitation.*

MEDICAL

> **OTHER LESS COMMON NURSING DIAGNOSES:** *High Risk for Disuse Syndrome;*
> *Impaired Social Interaction; Family Coping: Potential for growth;*
> *Body Image Disturbance; Altered Thought Processes*

ESSENTIAL DISCHARGE CRITERIA

- Shows no s/s of increased ICP
- Exhibits controlled bowel and bladder continence
- Performs prehospitalization level of ADL skills

- Parent/child demonstrates required care techniques; have list of s/s of complications to report; have follow-up appointments

NEAR-SIDS EVENT (Sudden Infant Death Syndrome)

NURSING DIAGNOSES	OUTCOME CRITERIA	INTERVENTIONS
1 Ineffective Breathing Pattern *r.t. near-SIDS of unknown etiology*	• Respirations WNL for age	• Assess RR, rhythm, and depth q2-4h • Provide continuous respiratory monitoring
	• Maintains O_2 sats > 95%	• Monitor O_2 sats continuously by pulse oximetry • Administer O_2 and ventilatory support as needed • Suction airway as needed
	• Is free of apneic events	• Monitor and record apneic events • Provide appropriate interventions to support breathing (tactile stimulation, positioning to maintain open airway, suctioning airway if necessary)
		RATIONALE: *Careful monitoring will alert caregiver to apneic episodes so appropriate interventions can be initiated.*
2 Fear *r.t. potential recurrence of event*	• Parents state their fears	• Assess and evaluate parents' support system and coping skills • Teach parents actions to take in case of apneic episode
	• Parents identify support network	• Refer parents to SIDS support group and other community services as appropriate • Provide counseling to family (in collaboration with interdisciplinary team)
		RATIONALE: *Self-confidence in care of their infant will optimize parents' relationship with their child and intervention in case of apneic spells.*

MEDICAL

NURSING DIAGNOSES	OUTCOME CRITERIA	INTERVENTIONS
3 Ineffective Family Coping: Compromised *r.t. sudden change in status of infant, stress related to near-death event, knowledge deficit*	• Parents verbalize concerns and fears	• Allow parents to verbalize fears and feelings related to near-death event
	• Parents demonstrate appropriate coping abilities	• Assess level of parents' anxiety, coping patterns, and skills • Refer parents to social worker and other support systems in the community
		RATIONALE: *Community and other supports will help minimize anxiety and fear and enhance the family's ability to cope with the near-death event.*
4 Knowledge Deficit *r.t. monitoring and diagnostic evaluation tests, home apnea monitoring, CPR*	• Parents have follow-up appointments scheduled	• Explain importance of follow-up appointments
	• Parents ask questions about causes of SIDS	• Explain how lab testing can establish the cause of near-SIDS event; provide facts on the causes of SIDS
	• Parents demonstrate - use of apnea monitor - infant CPR - appropriate interventions when apnea spells occur - monitoring requirements	• Provide infant CPR training and home apnea monitoring
		RATIONALE: *Appropriate monitoring and timely interventions can minimize potential devastating effects of apneic episodes.*

OTHER LESS COMMON NURSING DIAGNOSES:
Impaired Social Interaction; Impaired Gas Exchange

ESSENTIAL DISCHARGE CRITERIA

• Is free of apnea episodes

• Parents demonstrate ability to manage apnea and monitoring

• Parents demonstrate infant CPR

• Parents possess emergency phone numbers and verbalize plan for acute event

NURSING DIAGNOSES	OUTCOME CRITERIA	INTERVENTIONS
1 Fluid Volume Excess *r.t. intravascular to interstitial fluid shift associated with reduced plasma osmotic pressure*	• Shows decreasing edema	• Observe extremities, eyes for edema, puffiness qd • Measure abdominal girth at umbilicus qd
	• Body weight decreases toward pre-illness level	• Weigh daily, same time, same scale
	• Shows electrolytes WNL	• Monitor electrolytes
	• Shows normal postural BP, pulse	• Monitor VS, postural BP, pulses in extremities q4h
	• Has urinary sp. gr., protein WNL	• Assess urinary sp. gr. and protein q voiding
	• Restricts intake per orders	• Maintain strict and accurate I&O • Restrict salt, fluid per orders • Administer albumin IV, prednisone, diuretics, antihypertensives per orders; assess effects, side effects

RATIONALE: *Monitoring of the child's fluid status aids in evaluating and managing hydration.*

2 High Risk for Impaired Skin Integrity
 	
r.t. edema, immobility
	• Shows no signs of skin breakdown, irritation	• Inspect all skin surfaces for irritation, breakdown q4h
		• Protect skin
		  - turn, reposition q2h
		  - use pillows, soft padding to reduce pressure areas
		  - elevate edematous areas
		  - use soft cotton to separate skin surfaces and provide scrotal support
		  - use sheepskin, alternating air mattress
		  - wash, massage gently; use powder q4h
		  - perform passive ROM

RATIONALE: *Edematous skin is friable and especially prone to friction and breakdown. Muscle activity improves circulation.*

MEDICAL

NURSING DIAGNOSES	OUTCOME CRITERIA	INTERVENTIONS
3 Altered Nutrition: Less than body requirements *r.t. anorexia, albuminuria, ascites*	• Shows normalizing of body weight	• Weigh daily
	• Exhibits decreasing urinary albumin	• Test urinary albumin q4h
	• Eats 90% or more of meals	• Foster nutritional intake - serve 6 small meals qd - utilize parent, child, dietitian to plan diet - provide diet: high protein, high CHO; restrict Na - create pleasant, enjoyable meal times - include family in eating as a social occasion
		RATIONALE: *Children who are ill with nephrosis are likely to be anorexic. Special nutritional efforts need to be made.*
4 High Risk for Infection *r.t. immunosuppression*	• Shows no s/s of systemic infection - afebrile - VS, BP WNL - absence of cough, rigid abdomen, vomiting, diarrhea, rhinitis	• Monitor VS, BP q4-8h • Inspect all skin surfaces for irritation, breakdown q4h • Prevent infection - use strict hand-washing and universal precautions techniques - prohibit contact with ill staff, visitors - administer ordered antibiotics; assess effects - be aware of infection-masking by steroids
		RATIONALE: *Because nephrosis is treated with cortisone, the body's immune system is suppressed. Frequent monitoring for infection facilitates prompt antibiotic therapy.*

NURSING DIAGNOSES	OUTCOME CRITERIA	INTERVENTIONS
5 Diversional Activity Deficit *r.t. immobility, edema, fatigue*	• Plays quietly in bed	• Maintain bed rest, gradually increasing activities as edema subsides
	• Displays minimal fatigue from activities	• Prevent fatigue - offer quiet play activities - include parent/child in creating play activities - provide for naps, rest
		RATIONALE: *Because of edema and fatigue the child needs special attention to quiet, physically undemanding diversions.*
6 Altered Growth and Development *r.t. chronic illness*	• Displays age-appropriate developmental skills	• Assess developmental level; discuss assessment with parents • Assist parents to plan appropriate life and learning experiences to enhance growth and development
		RATIONALE: *Nephrosis is most common in children of ages 2-7, the years when much growth and development occurs. The frequent illnesses and hospitalizations can interrupt normal development.*
7 Altered Family Processes *r.t. chronic disruptions in family lifestyle*	• Parents express feelings, ask questions; take time away to attend to own ADLs	• Encourage feelings expression; reinforce positive coping behaviors
	• Parents participate in care	• Include family in care, diversional activities
	• Asserts self; verbalizes, displays personal pride	• Assist child to express feelings; assist with symbolic playing, drawing • Emphasize child's positive features, talents
	• Parents discuss specific ways to normalize lifestyle	• Discuss, problem-solve with parents about lifestyle management
		RATIONALE: *Because of the chronic nature of the disease, the family needs to be skilled in normalizing the family's and child's life.*

MEDICAL

NURSING DIAGNOSES	OUTCOME CRITERIA	INTERVENTIONS
8 **Knowledge Deficit** *r.t. home care of child associated with frequent recurrences of edema, complications*	• Parents discuss physiology of disease process, rationale for treatment	• Review physiology of disease
	• Parents perform urine testing, skin care, medications administration	• Explain, demonstrate required care techniques; obtain return demonstrations
	• Parents verbalize knowledge of s/s of complications: edema, weight gain, fever, skin infection, albuminuria	• Review, provide list of s/s to report to physician
	• Parents possess follow-up appointments	• Verify knowledge of follow-up appointments, community resources

RATIONALE: *Knowledgeable parents are likely to be successful in the child's many remissions and exacerbations.*

> ***OTHER LESS COMMON NURSING DIAGNOSES:***
> *Altered Tissue Perfusion; Impaired Social Interaction; Activity Intolerance*

ESSENTIAL DISCHARGE CRITERIA

- Shows urinary albumin within acceptable ranges
- Shows minimal edema
- Takes adequate amounts of food, fluids orally

- Shows dry, intact skin
- Parents verbalize, demonstrate knowledge of the treatment rationale, required care, s/s of complications, and follow-up appointments

NURSING DIAGNOSES	OUTCOME CRITERIA	INTERVENTIONS

1 High Risk for Injury (external)
 	
r.t. antineoplastic therapy: adverse effects related to bone marrow suppression, liver dysfunction, and/or renal insufficiency
	• Shows minimal adverse effects
	  - no anaphylactic reaction
	  - no s/s of infection
	  - normal functioning of cardiovascular, respiratory, central nervous, hematologic, gastrointestinal, hepatic, and genitourinary systems
		• Assess for contraindications to antineoplastic therapy
		  - hypersensitivity
		  - radiation therapy within 4 weeks prior
		  - severe bone marrow depression
		• Provide information and education regarding possible multi-system adverse reactions
		• Monitor, reduce severity of adverse effects
		  - document baseline assessment
		  - obtain baseline lab studies
		  - monitor VS for signs of infection
		  - ensure adequate nutrition
		  - monitor lab values
		  - monitor renal function
		  - monitor neuro VS

	• Parents reiterate, discuss prevention of complications	• Provide information regarding prevention of possible complications
		  - adequate follow-up care
		  - avoid crowded areas or potentially infectious persons
		  - drug interactions
		  - no live vaccines

	• Parents have list of reportable s/s	• Provide information regarding what s/s should be reported immediately
		  - fever
		  - chills, sweating
		  - diarrhea
		  - severe cough
		  - sore throat
		  - unusual bleeding
		  - burning on urination
		  - muscle cramps
		  - flu-like symptoms
		  - pain
		  - confusion, dizziness
		  - decreased urine output

RATIONALE: *Infection is a serious complication associated with chemotherapy administration due to bone marrow suppression. Liver dysfunction and renal insufficiency can occur with toxicity of chemotherapeutic agents.*

MEDICAL

NURSING DIAGNOSES	OUTCOME CRITERIA	INTERVENTIONS
2 High Risk for Fluid Volume Deficit *r.t. nausea and vomiting, decreased oral intake*	• Maintains circulating fluid volume WNL - urinary sp. gr. WNL - no pallor or cyanosis - VS WNL - capillary refill < 3 sec - good skin turgor	• Provide appealing forms of fluids for intake • Provide smaller, more frequent meals • Provide periods of rest prior to meals • Monitor urinary osmolality and sp. gr. • Assess VS, CRT q2-4h
	• Shows balanced I&O - weight remains stable for age	• Maintain strict I&O; weigh daily • Provide information about need to maintain a written record of fluid I&O and daily weights • Provide information about s/s of dehydration • Administer antiemetics as ordered
	• Shows blood work WNL	• Monitor serum electrolytes, BUN, creatinine, Hct, and Hb
		RATIONALE: *Dehydration can be associated with the nausea and vomiting that may be associated with antineoplastic agents. Decreased oral intake associated with the child's weakened condition may also contribute to dehydration.*
3 Altered Nutrition: Less than body requirements *r.t. anorexia secondary to chemotherapy, presence of abdominal mass*	• Takes, retains adequate nutrition - fats, carbohydrates, proteins - fluids	• Reduce contributing factors to anorexia - pain, fatigue - odors, nausea, vomiting • Provide appealing well-balanced meals, snacks • Encourage foods that stimulate the appetite and increase protein consumption; individualize to patient preference • Provide appealing snacks and meals that are appealing to child • Administer multivitamins and thiamine as ordered • Provide information about the importance of a balanced diet and improving nutrition status • Consult dietitian as needed

NURSING DIAGNOSES	OUTCOME CRITERIA	INTERVENTIONS
	• Maintains lab values WNL	• Monitor lab values such as CBC, serum cholesterol, electrolytes, and vitamins
	• Maintains intact oral mucosa	• Educate parents/child about importance of performing daily oral hygiene • Provide oral hygiene with prescribed mouthwash if stomatitis is present
		RATIONALE: *Chemotherapy-induced anorexia requires multiple strategies to enhance nutritional intake.*

4 Pain
 	
r.t. metastases to bone, compression of spinal cord, procedures
	• Displays, reports only minimal pain
	  - is not irritable
	  - does not guard or protect body
	  - displays relaxed body posture, facial expression
	  - has stable VS
		• Assess child's pain experience
		  - where it hurts
		  - intensity of pain
		  - what helps the pain
		  - parents' perspective of pain
		  - contributing factors: fear, loneliness, or anxiety
		• Provide information about pain and the treatment
		  - explain source of pain
		  - encourage parents to remain during procedures, if possible
		  - truthfully explain painful procedures
		  - explain use of narcotics, if applicable
		  - allow parents to verbalize feelings of helplessness about witnessing their child's pain

	• Parent/child verbalize understanding of pain relief measures	• Prepare child for painful procedures
		  - use terms that can be understood by the child
		  - introduce therapeutic play with instruments that will be used during the procedure
		  - encourage child to ask questions
		  - offer praise following the procedure
		• Minimize pain, anxiety during procedures
		  - minimize restraint time if used
		  - use distraction techniques
		  - provide privacy during painful procedures

MEDICAL

NURSING DIAGNOSES	OUTCOME CRITERIA	INTERVENTIONS

	• Verbalizes/displays comfort following analgesia	• Provide analgesics
		  - medicate prior to procedure or activity
		  - assess pain intensity
		  - use patient-controlled analgesia (PCA) when appropriate

		RATIONALE: *Pain related to primary site or metastases of the neuroblastoma can interfere with the child's and family's routines. Proper pain management, especially with invasive procedures, supports child's and family's maximum levels of functioning.*

> **OTHER LESS COMMON NURSING DIAGNOSES:** *Altered Urinary/Bowel Elimination; High Risk for Activity Intolerance; Altered Oral Mucous Membrane; Ineffective Family Coping: Compromised*

ESSENTIAL DISCHARGE CRITERIA

• Displays, reports adequate pain control

• Exhibits no s/s of multi-system complications

• Displays adequate hydration

• Takes, retains 80% of intake of a variety of nutrients

• Parents verbalize understanding of home care needs and list s/s to report to PCP

NURSING DIAGNOSES	OUTCOME CRITERIA	INTERVENTIONS

1 Pain

r.t. bone infection

- Verbalizes/displays no pain
  - reports sense of comfort
  - relaxed body posture, facial expressions
  - sleeps, naps at age-appropriate intervals

- Assess pain characteristics q2-4h using pediatric age-appropriate pain assessment scale
- Provide pain relief measures and monitor their effectiveness
  - analgesics q2-4h
  - support affected limb on pillows
  - use care in turning and moving
- Assure adequate sleep and rest
- Immobilize affected extremity
  - monitor the fit and position of immobilizing device q4h
  - maintain correct body alignment
  - splint/support affected part when movement is necessary
  - allow no weight bearing (high risk for pathologic fracture)
- Provide age-appropriate diversional activities

RATIONALE: *Using a consistent scale, language, and set of behaviors to assess pain will provide a more accurate assessment. A regular schedule for medication administration should be established to prevent severe pain. Proper use of the immobilizing device will enhance comfort.*

2 High Risk for Infection

r.t. presence of invasive device (catheter, irrigation tube/drain)

- Manifests no infection at the insertion site
  - VS WNL
  - WBC WNL
  - no change in appearance of skin around insertion site or adjacent structures

- Wash hands before and after contact with child
- Provide regular IV/tube site care using sterile technique
- Use sterile technique when accessing IV line
- Monitor VS q4h; notify physician if temperature is < 38°C (100.4°F)
- Observe site for swelling, warmth, or drainage
  - obtain sample of drainage for culturing
- Monitor lab data, WBC, and cultures

MEDICAL

NURSING DIAGNOSES	OUTCOME CRITERIA	INTERVENTIONS
	• Parent/child verbalize correct knowledge of home medication schedule	• Demonstrate the administration of IV medications using sterile technique (when applicable) • Demonstrate appropriate site care and related dressing changes • Instruct child/family in proper hand-washing technique
	• Identifies nutritional diet components to aid healing	• Describe a diet high in protein, calories, and vitamins
		RATIONALE: *Proper hand-washing and sterile technique reduce the transfer of infectious agents. Changes in vital signs, data, and site appearance may indicate the presence of infection.*
3 Impaired Physical Mobility *r.t. musculoskeletal impairment (infection of bone)*	• Exhibits dry, intact skin	• Inspect skin for intactness or reddened area with each position change • Keep bed as flat as possible
	• Exhibits undiminished muscle tone and joint function	• Utilize repositioning schedule; turn (or have child turn self) a minimum of q2h • Position child in neutral position with body weight evenly distributed - use pillows to support affected limbs • Provide ROM exercises on the nonaffected extremities a minimum of q shift • Encourage active ROM in the non-affected limbs a minimum of q shift, as tolerated
	• Participates in appropriate self-care activities	• If age-appropriate, involve child in planning daily routines • Allow child to participate in ADLs as able • Provide reading materials, toys, television, diversional activities and assist in their use, if necessary

NURSING DIAGNOSES	OUTCOME CRITERIA	INTERVENTIONS
	• Interacts with family and friends	• Keep child/family informed of events that will take place qd
		• Plan a special activity qd
		• Encourage parents/family to visit
		• Provide uninterrupted time for visits with family/friends
		• Encourage parent involvement in the child's care
		• Provide time for questions/answers
		• Encourage parents to bring in child's favorite toys

RATIONALE: *Frequent repositioning prevents prolonged pressure on the body surface areas. ROM exercise stimulates neuromuscular function. Play and involving the child in his/her care will reduce the monotony of immobility.*

NURSING DIAGNOSES	OUTCOME CRITERIA	INTERVENTIONS

4 **Knowledge Deficit**
 	
r.t. disease process, treatment plan, home maintenance management
	• Parent/child verbalize understanding of the disease process, the treatment plan, and home care needs
	  - recognize/report signs of infection
	  - describe the necessary activity restrictions
	  - describe the effects, side effects of oral/IV antibiotics
		• Discuss the disease process, the treatment plan, and home care needs

		• Identify knowledge deficits
		• Provide written information about the disease, treatment, medications
		• Prepare timetable for medication administration and drainage site care
		• Instruct in IV medication administration
		• Consult with dietitian for diet instructions
		• Refer to home health agency
		• Assist with follow-up appointments

RATIONALE: *Knowledgeable, competent parents are likely to provide safe, uneventful rehabilitation at home.*

> **OTHER LESS COMMON NURSING DIAGNOSES:** *Activity Intolerance; High Risk for Caregiver Role Strain; Constipation; High Risk for Impaired Skin Integrity; Social Isolation*

ESSENTIAL DISCHARGE CRITERIA

- Shows normal WBC
- Affirms adequate pain management
- Parent/child demonstrate understanding of home treatment plan

- Parents possess follow-up appointments and verbalize s/s to report to PCP

PNEUMONIA

NURSING DIAGNOSES	OUTCOME CRITERIA	INTERVENTIONS
1 Impaired Gas Exchange *r.t. ventilation perfusion imbalance secondary to mucus collection in alveoli*	• Shows decreasing evidence of respiratory distress, dyspnea	• Ausculate breath sounds q2-4h • Provide adequate oral or parenteral fluid intake per orders • Provide gentle tracheal suction as required • Provide O_2, cool mist as required • Assist to cough, deep breathe q1-2h • Elevate HOB or place child in infant seat • Perform chest physiotherapy q4h, per orders • Include parents in care and positioning
	• Exhibits normalizing, stable VS, normal skin color	• Monitor VS q2-4h; assess skin color
	• Exhibits normalizing ABGs; chest x-rays clearing	• Administer ordered antibiotics; assess effects, side effects • Monitor ABGs, chest x-rays • Monitor pulse oximeter q1-2h
		RATIONALE: *Frequent monitoring produces early detection of signs of respiratory compromise, prompting timely interventions.*
2 Hyperthermia *r.t. bacterial, viral invasion*	• Exhibits normalizing body temperature and VS	• Monitor temperature q2-4h
	• Verbalizes/displays evidence of reasonable comfort	• Provide ordered tepid sponges, cooling blanket for fever • Administer ordered analgesics, antipyretics; assess effects, side effects
		RATIONALE: *Keeping fever under control reduces metabolic demands and increases comfort.*

MEDICAL

NURSING DIAGNOSES	OUTCOME CRITERIA	INTERVENTIONS

3 Fluid Volume Deficit
 	
r.t. active fluid volume loss secondary to increased respiratory effort, dehydration secondary to hyperthermia
	• Manifests balanced I&O
	  - takes required fluids
	  - urinary output > 1 mL/kg/h
	  - normal urinary sp. gr.
	  - moist mucous membranes, good skin turgor, normal fontanel tension
		• Encourage frequent oral intake; include favorite fluids
		• Involve parents in finding ways to increase fluid intake
		• Administer IV fluids per orders
		• Monitor urinary output sp. gr. q8h
		• Assess mucous membranes, skin, fontanels q2-4h

		RATIONALE: *Monitoring and managing hydration offsets effects of RR and hyperthermia.*
4 Activity Intolerance *r.t. imbalance between O₂ supply and demand*	• Displays increased periods of alertness, play	• Provide toys, games within reach • Elevate HOB to decrease respiratory effort
	• Achieves/maintains normal patterns of sleeping, napping	• Plan care activities to ensure uninterrupted rest periods • Maintain quiet environment • Reposition q2h for position of comfort • Involve parents in promoting rest
		RATIONALE: *Paced activity and O₂ therapy minimize imbalance of O₂ supply and demand.*
5 Knowledge Deficit *r.t. inexperience, fear of recurrence*	• Parents discuss pathophysiology of disease process, probable cause, treatment rationale, expected course, potential for recurrence	• Explain pneumonia: pathophysiology, treatment rationale, prognosis • Involve parents in providing care and comfort measures
	• Parents verbalize understanding of signs to report to physician: fever, cough, dyspnea, pallor, cyanosis	• Describe/provide parents with a list of signs of complications
	• Parents discuss ways to prevent recurrence	• Discuss specific methods of prevention based upon most likely precipitating factors in this episode of illness

NURSING DIAGNOSES	OUTCOME CRITERIA	INTERVENTIONS
	• Parents list medications: effects, side effects, dosage, and how to administer	• Teach medications, effects, side effects, route of administration, dosage
	• Parents verbalize knowledge of expected follow-up with physician	• Verify that parents know about expected follow-up
		RATIONALE: *Knowledgeable, competent parents are likely to provide for a safe, uneventful recovery.*

MEDICAL

OTHER LESS COMMON NURSING DIAGNOSES: *Ineffective Airway Clearance; Altered Nutrition: Less than body requirements; Ineffective Breathing Pattern; Fatigue*

ESSENTIAL DISCHARGE CRITERIA

• Is afebrile

• Tolerates ADLs without respiratory distress

• Takes food, fluids qs

• Parents verbalize knowledge of home care and expected follow-up

POISONING

NURSING DIAGNOSES	OUTCOME CRITERIA	INTERVENTIONS
1 Ineffective Breathing Pattern *r.t. depression of respiratory center secondary to toxic ingestants*	• RR, rhythm, and depth are WNL for age	• Assess RR, rhythm, and depth q2-4h
	• Maintains O$_2$ sats > 95%	• Monitor O$_2$ sats continuously by pulse oximetry • Administer O$_2$ and ventilatory support as needed • Suction airway as needed
		RATIONALE: *Many ingestants cause respiratory depression; therefore, airway management is essential.*
2 Decreased Cardiac Output *r.t. depression of circulatory system secondary to toxic ingestants*	• Achieves, maintains stable vital signs WNL	• Assess vital signs qh • Place on continuous cardiopulmonary monitor • Monitor ECG for rhythm disturbance such as bradycardia, PVC
	• Maintains good perfusion with capillary refill < 3 sec	• Assess skin perfusion q2-4h
		RATIONALE: *Many ingestants cause circulatory depression and dysrhythmias, therefore vital signs should be monitored closely to prevent altered tissue perfusion.*
3 High Risk for Fluid Volume Deficit *r.t. excessive losses secondary to treatments that decrease absorption and increase elimination of ingestant*	• Maintains balanced I&O	• Give IV fluids as ordered • Maintain accurate I&O
	• Loses no more than 2% of weight daily	• Weigh daily at same time on same scale
	• Maintains good perfusion with capillary refill < 3 sec	• Assess skin perfusion q2-4h • Administer medications to decrease absorption or increase elimination as ordered by physician
		RATIONALE: *Interventions that promote elimination of ingested poison from the system cause fluid loss. Monitoring and management of hydration are required for recovery.*

NURSING DIAGNOSES	OUTCOME CRITERIA	INTERVENTIONS
4 High Risk for Injury *r.t. disorientation*	• Exhibits no signs of injury	• Assess LOC q2-4h, or as indicated • Orient to place and time q2-4h when appropriate • Keep side rails up at all times and bed in the low position • Apply soft restraints to wrists and ankles as needed • Explain safety concerns to parents or guardian • Be alert for seizure activity
		RATIONALE: *Monitoring LOC and instituting safety precautions protect child from physical injury during periods of disorientation or seizure/activity*
5 High Risk for Poisoning *r.t. individual and environmental factors*	• Parents discuss how this episode may have been prevented; identify specific safety measures to institute	• Instruct parents to store all cleaning products out of reach of children with safety locks on all cabinets • Instruct parents to keep all medications out of reach of children • Instruct parents not to refer to medications as candy • Encourage parents to check that household plants are not poisonous • Encourage parents to check basements and garage to be sure that all paints, solvents, and fertilizers are out of reach of children • Encourage parents or guardians to have Ipecac at home • Provide parents with the number for the local poison control center
		RATIONALE: *The solution to the problem of childhood poisonings lies in prevention.*

MEDICAL

207

> **OTHER LESS COMMON NURSING DIAGNOSES:** *Altered Nutrition: Less than body requirements; Altered Family Processes; Ineffective Family Coping: Compromised; Knowledge Deficit*
> *Other nursing diagnoses are dependent on the type of poisoning and require treatments specific to that ingestant*

ESSENTIAL DISCHARGE CRITERIA

- Shows adequate oxygenation, easy respirations

- Exhibits no symptoms attributable to ingestant

- Parents identify preventative measures to safeguard the child at home

- Parents verbalize plans for home care and list s/s to report to PCP

QUADRIPLEGIA, SPINAL CORD INJURY

NURSING DIAGNOSES	OUTCOME CRITERIA	INTERVENTIONS
1 Impaired Gas Exchange *r.t. ineffective airway clearance secondary to mucus secretions, tracheostomy*	• Exhibits normal VS	• Monitor VS q2-4h
	• Exhibits normal ABGs	• Monitor ABGs; report changes outside of parameters
	• Displays no cyanosis, pallor, dyspnea, restlessness, tachypnea	• Monitor, manage respiratory support - assess respiratory status q2-4h; - assess ability to cough - use cardio/apnea alarm - perform clapping, postural drainage; involve respiratory therapist in plans - suction prn - force fluids per orders
		RATIONALE: *Close monitoring produces prompt management. Clapping, postural drainage, and suction produce clearing of collected secretions.*
2 High Risk for Injury (internal) *r.t. postural hypotension*	• Sits up, stands with help without feeling faint	• Monitor postural hypotension - assess BP before and after sitting, standing until s/s absent - assess for dizziness during elevation of head
	• Experiences no falls, near-falls during transfers	• Reduce potential effects of postural hypotension - gradually increase incline of upper body - gradually increase sitting time - use wraps, corsets before sitting, standing
		RATIONALE: *Autonomic dysfunction may produce massive vasodilation and pooling of blood below level of injury, causing postural hypotension. Gradual position change distributes blood flow more evenly, reducing fainting, dizziness.*

MEDICAL

NURSING DIAGNOSES	OUTCOME CRITERIA	INTERVENTIONS

3 High Risk for Injury (external)
 	
r.t. falls associated with muscle spasms
	• Experiences no falls or near-falls when transferring, standing
	
	• Exhibits decreasing frequency of muscle spasms
		• Protect when transferring, sitting, standing
		
		• Assess frequency, duration of spasms
		  - identify precipitating stimuli
		  - administer ordered antispasmodics: assess effects, side effects
		
		RATIONALE: *Reducing precipitating stimuli and providing physical support for moving help to prevent falls. Antispasmodics reduce effects of precipitating stimuli.*

4 High Risk for Injury (internal)
 	
r.t. thrombophlebitis associated with immobility, impaired circulation
	• Shows negative Homan's sign
	
	• Has no localized heat, redness, swelling
	
	• Shows no cyanosis, respiratory distress
		• Assess Homan's sign bid
		
		• Observe for tenderness, swelling of calves, bid
		
		• Prevent, detect embolism
		  - reposition q2h
		  - elevate legs; use elastic wraps (feet to groin)
		  - keep feet dorsiflexed
		  - observe for cyanosis, respiratory distress each time in room
		
		RATIONALE: *Repositioning, elastic wraps, and dorsiflexion reduce venous pooling of blood in large veins of legs. Early detection of respiratory distress or s/s of venous tenderness produces prompt medical intervention.*

5 High Risk for Injury (physical)
 	
r.t. joint contractures associated with immobility, spasticity
	• Displays full or baseline ROM	• Prevent contractures
		  - passive ROM all joints q4h
		  - provide splints for functional positioning
		  - use high-top tennis shoes for foot drop prevention
		  - involve physical therapist in plans

NURSING DIAGNOSES	OUTCOME CRITERIA	INTERVENTIONS
		RATIONALE: *Thorough and frequent ROM and other physical therapy exercises maintain baseline joint mobility. Splinting and functional positioning counteract the effects of spasticity.*

6 High Risk for Impaired Skin Integrity
 	
r.t. immobility; impaired circulation
	• Displays clear, intact skin	• Protect skin
		  - reposition q2h
		  - increase chair to tid, prn
		  - inspect skin q4h
		  - massage bony prominences q4h
		  - use sheepskin, eggcrate, footboard

		RATIONALE: *Venous pooling reduces flow of O_2 and cell nutrients and, combined with pressure, produces skin breakdown.*
7 Self-Esteem Disturbance *r.t. physical, biological, perceptual, psychosocial limitations*	• Makes positive self-assertions	• Give positive feedback for strengths; involve family
	• Performs own ADLs to maximum of ability	• Involve in own ADLs
	• Maintains eye contact	• Encourage self-expression
		RATIONALE: *Positive support maximumizes the ability to perform self-care and fosters feelings of self-worth. The child internalizes positive verbal feedback, which also enhances feelings of self-worth.*

8 Altered Urinary Elimination
 	
r.t. sensory motor impairment
	• Has no urinary retention	• Monitor, prevent urinary retention
		  - palpate bladder q6h for distention
		  - perform ordered intermittent catheterization, bladder tapping, Credé, thigh stroking

		RATIONALE: *Loss of nervous function increases the potential for retention.*

MEDICAL

NURSING DIAGNOSES	OUTCOME CRITERIA	INTERVENTIONS
9 **High Risk for Infection** *r.t. urinary retention*	• Shows no s/s urinary infection - is afebrile - has clear amber urine with no foul smell	• Monitor s/s of urinary infection - monitor VS q4h - inspect urine for cloudiness, odor
		RATIONALE: *Urinary status increased the rise of bacterial proliferation.*
10 **Bowel Incontinence** *r.t. neuromuscular impairment*	• Has bowel movement q1-3d - soft, formed stool (no hard-formed stool, no diarrhea) - bowel sounds present - no abdominal distention	• Establish bowel routine per hospital protocol - maintain balanced I&O - encourage fluids - auscultate bowel sounds q4-6h - palpate abdomen for distention q4-6h
		RATIONALE: *Neuromuscular impairment alters bowel function and necessitates regular attention to bowel care.*
11 **Altered Nutrition: Less than body requirements** *r.t. anorexia associated with immobility*	• Has body weight within 20% of ideal for height, frame	• Weigh daily
	• Manifests normal Hb, Hct	• Monitor Hb, Hct
	• Takes at least 90% of required nutrients	• Maintain required intake - offer preferred foods high in protein, vitamins, minerals - encourage high fluid intake - include child, family in meal planning - create pleasant mealtimes
		RATIONALE: *A combination of highly nutritious foods, fluids, preferred foods, and pleasant, social mealtime enhances nutritional intake.*

NURSING DIAGNOSES	OUTCOME CRITERIA	INTERVENTIONS

12 Altered Growth and Development
 	
r.t. neurologic impairment, limited stimuli, limited social activity
	• Performs age-appropriate developmental tasks within limits of disability	• Monitor, stimulate developmental performance
		  - assess developmental level
		  - provide organized program of stimuli, activity
		  - do not overstimulate
		  - encourage normalcy in ADL, clothing
		  - teach parents about growth and development even under conditions of quadriplegia

	• Interacts with staff, family, peers	• Encourage room decoration, peer interaction
		RATIONALE: *Maximizing normal activities and social interactions enhances mastery of growth and development tasks.*
13 Knowledge Deficit *r.t. providing for multiple demands of quadriplegic child*	• Parent/child assist with care (as appropriate); demonstrate required care skills	• Involve parents and child (if age-appropriate) in care; demonstrate home care skills
	• Parent/child discuss s/s of complications: fever, skin breakdown, contractures, cloudy urine, constipation, diarrhea, lethargy, pallor, hot and tender area of extremity	• Describe potential complications; provide list
	• Parent/child are involved in appropriate support group	• Refer to support group(s) as appropriate
	• Parents verbalize knowledge of follow-up appointments	• Refer to discharge coordinator for home care evaluation, planning; verify possession of follow-up appointments

MEDICAL

NURSING DIAGNOSES	OUTCOME CRITERIA	INTERVENTIONS
	• Parent/child demonstrate ability to perform ADLs under controlled conditions	• Prior to discharge, child goes home on 24-h pass (times 1-2 as necessary) with team leader visits bid - assess home environment for necessary changes to enhance caregiving - parents take complete control for limited time with opportunity to discuss care with team upon return to hospital - necessary changes can be made with input from team

RATIONALE: *Knowledgeable, competent parents and family are likely to successfully manage the long-term care requirements of the child.*

OTHER LESS COMMON NURSING DIAGNOSES: *Social Isolation; Altered Family Processes; High Risk for Caregiver Role Strain; Altered Growth and Development*

ESSENTIAL DISCHARGE CRITERIA

• Maintains full or baseline ROM

• Has controlled bladder, bowel continence

• Performs own ADL within limits of ability

• Parents demonstrate required care skills and understand s/s of complications

• Parents possess follow-up appointment(s), identify required sources of support, assistance

RESPIRATORY DISTRESS

NURSING DIAGNOSES	OUTCOME CRITERIA	INTERVENTIONS
1 Impaired Gas Exchange *r.t. pulmonary compromise, infectious process*	• Achieves/maintains adequate oxygenation; shows no evidence of - abnormal ABGs - nasal flaring - expiratory grunt - retractions	• Administer O_2 via method appropriate for type of respiratory compromise • Monitor/observe for changes in respiratory status • Monitor/observe child's response to mechanical ventilation • Observe for apnea, nasal flaring, expiratory grunt, cyanosis • Monitor ABGs as appropriate • Position child to allow for maximal lung expansion • Suction as needed • Minimize noxious environmental stimuli • Monitor response and side effects of prescribed medications **RATIONALE:** *Early detection/management of deteriorating respiratory status improves chances that an infant will be able to breathe and maintain optimum blood gas measurements without ventilator assistance.*
2 Ineffective Breathing Pattern *r.t. airway obstruction, neurologic compromise*	• Maintains effective breathing pattern - satisfactory rate, depth, rhythm of respirations - adequate oxygenation - stable or improved lab values	• Constantly monitor and observe child's response to ventilatory support • Provide continuous cardiorespiratory monitoring • Ausculate heart sounds, breath sounds q2h; report deviations **RATIONALE:** *Constant monitoring assures early detection and management of complications.*

MEDICAL

NURSING DIAGNOSES	OUTCOME CRITERIA	INTERVENTIONS
3 Altered Nutrition: Less than body requirements *r.t. respiratory distress, feeding intolerance*	• Attains and maintains normal nutritional status as evidenced by weight gain	• Weigh daily, same scale • Maintain caloric intake through intravenous, TPN, or gavage feeding
	• Maintains normal blood sugar levels	• Monitor for hypoglycemia, especially during stress

	• Maintains balanced I&O
	  - urinary output 1-3 mL/kg/h
	  - urinary sp. gr. WNL
		• Provide 80-120 kcal/kg/24h
		• Maintain strict I&O, monitor sp. gr. q2-4h

	• Remains free of signs of GI complications
	  - stable abdominal girth
	  - normal elimination pattern
	  - tolerances of enteral feeding
		• Monitor for signs of gastrointestinal complications
		  - distress
		  - constipation/diarrhea
		  - frequent vomiting
		• Measure residual prior to gavage feedings

		RATIONALE: *Maintenance of sufficient nutrition provides energy and helps to compensate for the high metabolic demands of respiratory distress.*
4 Altered Parenting *r.t. situational crisis associated with complex care requirements*	• Parents display appropriate parent-child attachment as demonstrated by parental behaviors and verbalization, responses of infant	• Encourage parent-child interaction • Provide developmentally appropriate auditory, tactile, and visceral stimulation
	• Parents are actively involved and assist in planning and giving care, as appropriate	• Encourage family to participate as possible in care • Encourage parental decision-making when appropriate • Allow parents to verbalize concerns and questions regarding illness, equipment, and care being provided • Encourage family to plan for long-term follow-up, as appropriate
		RATIONALE: *Parental and infant attachment fosters positive parenting behaviors.*

OTHER LESS COMMON NURSING DIAGNOSES: *Altered Growth and Development; High Risk for Infection; Sensory/Perceptual Alterations; Knowledge Deficit (parents); Altered Tissue Perfusion (cardiopulmonary)*

ESSENTIAL DISCHARGE CRITERIA

- Shows easy respirations on room air
- Takes and tolerates 90% of prescribed feedings
- Parents demonstrate effective care skills, display appropriate bonding behaviors
- Parents possess follow-up appointments and lists s/s to report to PCP

REYE SYNDROME

NURSING DIAGNOSES	OUTCOME CRITERIA	INTERVENTIONS

1 Altered Tissue Perfusion (cerebral) *r.t. cerebral edema, increased ICP*	• Experiences prompt identification of neurologic changes
	  - fatigue, restlessness, irritability
	  - lethargy, vomiting
	  - elevated liver enzymes
	  - posturing (decorticate, decerebrate)
	  - pupillary changes
	  - seizures, coma
		• Monitor changes in neuro status qh

	• Maintains adequate cerebral perfusion
	  - cerebral perfusion pressure > 50 mmHg
	  - VS WNL
	  - ICP 4-15 mmHg
		• Monitor, control ICP qh
		  - elevate HOB 30°
		  - keep head in neutral alignment
		  - hyperventilate (per order) if ICP > 20 mmHg
		• Monitor VS and central venous pressure q1-2h

	• Is alert, oriented to person, place, and time	• Assess level of responsiveness q1-2h

	• Sustains no seizure-related injuries	• Maintain seizure precautions
		  - O$_2$ and suction at bedside
		  - reduce stimuli

	• Maintains body temperature WNL	• Monitor temperature (axillary/rectal) qh
		  - sponge bath
		  - use thermal blanket for heating or cooling

		RATIONALE: *Frequent monitoring prompts early identification and treatment of altered cerebral perfusion.*

2 Altered Tissue Perfusion (systemic) *r.t. altered electrolytes and coagulopathies secondary to liver dysfunction*	• Experiences prompt identification of risk factors
	  - serum ammonia > 80 mg/dL
	  - increased amino acids
	  - elevated SGOT, SGPT
	  - hypoglycemia
		• Monitor lab values q8h
		  - liver enzymes
		  - electrolytes
		  - serum osmolarity
		  - glucose
		• Administer fluids and electrolytes per orders

	• Maintains CVP at 5 mmHg • Has warm skin with instant capillary refill < 3 sec	• Monitor/maintain CVP q2h - administer IV fluids as ordered

NURSING DIAGNOSES	OUTCOME CRITERIA	INTERVENTIONS
	• Shows ABGs WNL	• Monitor ABGs q8h
		RATIONALE: *Frequent monitoring for evidence of altered systemic perfusion prompts timely intervention.*
3 High Risk for Injury (internal bleeding) *r.t. altered coagulation factors*	• Shows clotting factors WNL - PT, PTT, platelets	• Monitor lab values for clotting factors q8h

	• Exhibits no s/s of bleeding
	  - stool, urine, vomitus negative
	    for occult blood
	  - no frank bleeding
	  - no bruising or petechiae
		• Monitor/control s/s of bleeding
		  - urine check for blood q8h
		  - guaiac stool, vomitus q8h
		  - inspect for bruises, frank bleeding
		  - administer blood products as
		    ordered
		  - administer Vitamin K as ordered

		RATIONALE: *Frequent monitoring prompts early identification and management of bleeding.*

4 High Risk for Fluid Volume Deficit
 	
r.t. vomiting, altered renal perfusion
	• Is well hydrated
	  - moist mucous membranes
	  - elastic skin turgor
	  - tears
	  - normal fontanel tension
		• Assess hydration status q2h

	• Maintains balanced I&O
	  - no weight fluctuations
	  - urine output WNL for weight
	  - sp. gr. WNL
		• Maintain strict I&O
		  - administer IV fluids per order
		  - monitor urine output, sp. gr
		  - weigh daily

	• Experiences no vomiting	• Slowly advance from NPO to regular diet
		RATIONALE: *Constant evaluation and management of fluid balance are required to augment renal function.*

MEDICAL

NURSING DIAGNOSES	OUTCOME CRITERIA	INTERVENTIONS

5 Anxiety
r.t. sudden onset of illness, severity of illness, procedures, hospitalization, unknown prognosis/sequelae
	• Exhibits minimal anxiety
	  - BP, pulse, respirations WNL
	  - relates an increase in physiological and psychological comfort
	  - parents express feelings of concern
		• Monitor for evidence of anxiety
		• Provide consistent caregivers
		  - offer support and reassurance
		  - encourage expression of worry, grief
		  - initiate supportive services if needed
		• Explain procedures to child/parent
		• Provide consistent explanations and updates on progress

	• Parents participate in care of child	• Encourage parents' participation in care
		  - touch, stroke, talk to, sing to
		  - bring from home a favorite toy or security object
		  - engage child in quiet play if appropriate

		RATIONALE: *Giving information about a procedure helps to decrease anxiety. Familiar objects help to reduce anxiety.*
6 Knowledge Deficit *r.t. lack of experience with disease process, home care of child*	• Parents discuss s/s of Reye Syndrome	• Instruct parents about s/s of Reye Syndrome, its treatment and usual cause
	• Parents verbalize knowledge of products containing salicylates	• Provide parents with list of over-the-counter products which may contain hidden salicylates

	• Parents demonstrate required care of child	• Include parents in care techniques
		  - demonstrate home care requirements
		  - identify community resources for support and assistance

		RATIONALE: *Knowledge of this information eases anxiety and increases parents' confidence in the child's recovery and ability to provide rehabilitative care.*

OTHER LESS COMMON NURSING DIAGNOSES: *Sensory/Perceptual Alterations; Altered Nutrition: Less than body requirements; Altered Urinary Elimination; Impaired Skin Integrity; Altered Growth and Development; Altered Family Processes; Altered Thought Processes*

ESSENTIAL DISCHARGE CRITERIA

- Demonstrates orientation to person, place, and time
- Maintains respiratory pattern, BP, HR, and temperature WNL
- Exhibits no s/s of increased ICP
- Takes adequate fluids and nutrition
- Parents demonstrate ability to care for child and list s/s to report to PCP

MEDICAL

SEIZURE DISORDERS

NURSING DIAGNOSES	OUTCOME CRITERIA	INTERVENTIONS
1 Ineffective Breathing Patterns *r.t. neuromuscular impairment secondary to seizure activity*	• Maintains adequate ventilation and oxygenation during seizures - maintains O_2 sats > 95% - exhibits no cyanosis - exhibits no tachypnea, retractions, apnea	• Place suction canister and appropriate size suction catheter at bedside with O_2 set-up on admission • Monitor pulse oximetry if child is at high risk for seizure activity
	• Is free from hypoxia-related injury	• Protect child during seizure activity - turn child to side-lying to maintain patent airway and allow secretions to drool - provide O_2 blowby with mask - suction oral secretions prn • do not insert a tongue blade or other objects; this may occlude the child's airway - assess respiratory status continuously, especially after administering anticonvulsive medications IV - insert an NG tube if s/s of decreased LOC
		RATIONALE: *These interventions maintain patent airway, provide for adequate oxygenation, and prevent aspiration and respiratory stress leading to respiratory failure.*
2 High Risk for Injury (cerebral) *r.t. anoxia secondary to seizure*	• Sustains no further brain insult resulting from seizure activity - exhibits LOC at pre-seizure status - remains in post-ictal state for expected duration - exhibits intact pupillary responses and reflexes - exhibits minimal side effects from prn and maintenance anticonvulsant medications	• Maintain IV access • Know patient-specific safe dose for anticonvulsants • Watch for drowsiness, nystagmus, slurred speech, GI upset, stomatitis • Keep resuscitative equipment available for ventilatory support
	• Parents demonstrate required care knowledge and techniques	• Instruct parents on how to manage care • Explain how to calibrate maintenance doses • Encourage parents to give medications with meals

NURSING DIAGNOSES	OUTCOME CRITERIA	INTERVENTIONS
		RATIONALE: *Monitoring and calibrating child's responses to medication are essential to his/her safety. Parents also need to know how to manage pharmacological seizure control.*
3 High Risk for Injury (external) *r.t. neuromuscular, perceptual, cognitive impairment secondary to seizure activity*	• Sustains no injuries during seizures	• Use padded side rails • Loosen clothing at neck • Remove sharp, hard objects from bed • If standing or sitting in a chair during a seizure, slide gently to the floor and position side-lying, with padding under the head • Do not attempt to restrain or use force • Do not attempt to put anything in child's mouth • Stay with child • Protect child's head from injury
	• Parent/child share their knowledge and success with pre- and post-seizure safety precautions	• Assesses parent's, child's knowledge of care during seizures - prodromal s/s - characteristics of seizure activity - safety measures to be taken by child or adolescent (swimming, public transportation, driving)
	• Parent/child identify ways to improve management and safety in future	• Assist family to improve skills, knowledge
		RATIONALE: *Safety measures, protection, and anticipatory preparation reduce incidence of injuries from seizures.*

MEDICAL

NURSING DIAGNOSES	OUTCOME CRITERIA	INTERVENTIONS

4 Knowledge Deficit
 	
r.t. disease process, medications, injury prevention
	• Parents verbalize knowledge of disease process and of medication administration	• Teach parent/child about seizures
		  - definitions of a seizure and causes
		  - actions to be taken during a seizure
		  - drug names, times, amounts, purpose, and side effects
		  - emphasize need for consistent drug therapy regardless of the presence or absence of seizures
		  - give the child honest and age-appropriate information
		  - encourage parents to provide for optimal development, not over-protection

	• Parents identify needs and note specific helpful resources	• Provide and identify available community services
		  - epilepsy parent support groups
		  - National Epilepsy Foundation

	• Parents possess appointments for required follow-up care	• Alert school nurse and teachers regarding diagnosis and what to do during a seizure
		RATIONALE: *Parental/child noncompliance with medications and nontreatment of fevers can precipitate status epilepticus. Parental noncompliance is usually related to poor understanding rather than carelessness or lack of concern.*

> ***OTHER LESS COMMON NURSING DIAGNOSES:*** *Alteration in Nutrition: Less than body requirements; Altered Family Processes; Noncompliance (parental); Anxiety (family); Body Image Disturbance*

ESSENTIAL DISCHARGE CRITERIA

- Achieves, maintains seizure control
- Maintains adequate ventilation

- Parent/child demonstrate competence with safety precautions and seizure management
- Parent/child demonstrate knowledge of safe medication administration

NURSING DIAGNOSES	OUTCOME CRITERIA	INTERVENTIONS
1 Altered Tissue Perfusion (cerebral, cardio-pulmonary, splenic, renal, peripheral) *r.t. microcirculation associated with sickling of RBCs, decreased O2-carrying capacity of blood*	• Experiences adequate/normal tissue perfusion - normal, stable BP, VS - no increase in spleen size - no decrease in Hb, Hct - no abdominal distention, left-sided abdominal pain, or vomiting - capillary refill < 3 sec - warm extremities - cyanosis absent, decreasing - no reports or displays of pain, dizziness, weakness, restlessness, chest pain, altered LOC, orthostatic VS	• Monitor BP, VS; assess orthostatic VS q4h prn • Assess spleen size; monitor Hb, Hct for decreases • Assess for abdominal distention, left-sided abdominal pain, vomiting, shock • Assess capillary refill time; assess lips, mucous membranes, nail beds for cyanosis q4h • Monitor LOC; observe for pain, dizziness, weakness, restlessness, chest pain, altered LOC
	• Experiences safe blood transfusions	• Monitor blood transfusions to avoid fluid overload - monitor VS - infuse slowly (5-10 mL/kg) • Administer blood products per institutional standards
		RATIONALE: *Frequent monitoring permits early detection of s/s of inadequate tissue perfusion. Early detection results in prompt medical and nursing management. Blood transfusions increase the O2-carrying capacity of the blood.*
2 High Risk for Activity Intolerance *r.t. compromised tissue oxygenation*	• Tolerates moderate activity without cyanosis or shortness of breath	• Monitor and manage exertional dyspnea - report chest pain - keep O2 at bedside; administer for cyanosis; assess effects - use O2 only as prescribed - encourage bed rest; gradually introduce activity as tolerated - schedule care to maximize rest periods - closely monitor child during activity
	• Parent, child identify those activities that can be tolerated during a crisis	• Involve parent/child in activity decisions • Refer to child life specialist to identify alternative activities
		RATIONALE: *Careful balancing of activity and rest maximizes oxygenation of vital body centers. Hypoxia triggers erythropoeisis.*

MEDICAL

NURSING DIAGNOSES	OUTCOME CRITERIA	INTERVENTIONS
3 Fluid Volume Deficit *r.t. low fluid intake, impaired renal function*	• Is adequately hydrated - moist mucous membranes, good skin turgor, normal fontanel tension, tears - serum electrolytes WNL - urinary output of at least 1 mL/kg/h - maintains weight at pre-illness level; without significant fluctuation - capillary refill < 3 secs; intact peripheral pulses	• Inspect mucous membranes, skin, fontanels, corneas q4h • Monitor BP q4h as required • Monitor electrolytes • Monitor urinary output within 2h of fluid therapy • Weigh daily • Assess CRT and peripheral pulses
	• Takes prescribed amount of fluids (1½ times fluid maintenance requirement)	• Monitor, manage I&O - calculate child's fluid maintenance requirements - force fluids unless contraindicated - frequently offer favorite, colorful fluids (jello, popsicles, slurpees made with slightly melted popsicles and 7-Up) - use interesting straws, glasses, bottles, etc. - administer ordered fluid infusions at maintenance rate; assess effects
		RATIONALE: *Renal function may be impaired as part of disease process, which requires hydration vigilance. Note that urinary sp. gr. and quantity of output may be inaccurate indicators of hydration if renal function is impaired. Body weight is the best indicator of fluid loss or retention.*
4 High Risk for Infection *r.t. pneumonia secondary to occluded pulmonary arterioles, limited splenic filtering of bacteria*	• Becomes afebrile within 48-72h of antibiotic therapy	• Administer antibiotics as ordered • Monitor body temperature q2h • Provide ordered antipyretics, tepid sponging to control fever
	• Displays no s/s of respiratory distress - retractions, dyspnea, flaring - cough - tachycardia - lethargy, pallor - tachypnea	• Assess respiratory status q2-4h

NURSING DIAGNOSES	OUTCOME CRITERIA	INTERVENTIONS
	• Shows decrease in pulmonary mucus secretions	• Assist with coughing, deep breathing q2h
	• Parents discuss ways to minimize risk of respiratory infection	• Instruct parents how to minimize risks of infection • Restrict contacts with staff, visitors with URI • Assess immunization status of child, siblings; recommend updates
		RATIONALE: *Because of possible occlusion of arterioles, maintaining O$_2$ sats at a safe level is important to reduce chance of infection. Limiting O$_2$ needs and preventing infection through immunization and restricted contacts with URI are essential.*
5 Impaired Gas Exchange *r.t. stasis of RBCs, vaso-occlusion, lung infarctions*	• Exhibits optimal oxygenation of tissues - clear breath sounds - normal color - activity tolerance	• Assess respirations, breath sounds, pain, oxygenation • Identify factors contributing to decreased oxygenation (infection, emotional stress, physical activity) • Provide humidified O$_2$ as prescribed • Position for comfort and optimal oxygenation • Maintain O$_2$ sats > 95%
	• Parents describe, discuss preventative strategies against vaso-occlusive crisis	• Include parents in discussion about the physiology of vaso-occlusion; teach preventative strategies
		RATIONALE: *Maximize tissue oxygenation and minimize negative effects of tissue hypoxia.*

MEDICAL

NURSING DIAGNOSES	OUTCOME CRITERIA	INTERVENTIONS
6 Pain *r.t. tissue hypoxia secondary to vaso-occlusive crisis*	• Experiences sustained comfort levels - behaviors are consistent with comfort - pain controlled with oral medications - sleeps, naps WNL for age - laughs, smiles, talks, maintain's eye contact	• Assess pain, including intensity, location, factors contributing to pain crisis • Assess effectiveness of current pain control plan • Monitor response to pain management techniques using a pain scale • Administer medications according to sickle cell pain protocol
	• Parent/child demonstrate, discuss proper pain management: medications, treatments, comfort measures; distraction, relaxation, rest	• Enlist family/child to choose and implement nonpharmacologic modes of pain management - positioning - heat - distraction - relaxation techniques - rest - hydration • Teach rationale of pharmacologic pain management
		RATIONALE: *Consistent pain management techniques are required for sustained comfort. Sustained comfort reduces O_2, metabolic demands.*
7 Altered Growth and Development *r.t. chronic illness*	• Makes positive self-reports; asserts self, make eye contact	• Allow parents/child to express feelings, fears
	• Laughs, talks, initiates interactions with staff, peers	• Encourage a near-normal lifestyle, school studies within hospital
	• Accomplishes age-appropriate developmental tasks	• Provide developmentally appropriate activities • Give positive feedback for efforts • Encourage child, adolescent to assume appropriate responsibility for self
	• Parents show love, holding, touching; participate in care	• Encourage parents to hold, cuddle, touch, stroke child
	• Parents set limits; set expectations	• Encourage set limits, expectations as with any child
		RATIONALE: *Knowledgeable, competent parents are likely to provide experiences and support that foster normal growth and development.*

NURSING DIAGNOSES	OUTCOME CRITERIA	INTERVENTIONS
8 Ineffective Family Coping: Potential for growth *r.t. the expert support, counseling that is available to a family in crisis*	• Family/child display strong coping strategies - express feelings, fears - make positive, self-affirming statements - seek help, support	• Identify primary patient care coordinator for patient/family • Refer to local support groups • Refer to social worker **RATIONALE:** *Child/family will be better able to cope if dependable support system is available.*
9 High Risk for Injury *r.t. physical activity*	• Parent/child identify activities to be avoided	• Teach which activities are high risk for accidents; discuss avoidance techniques • Refer to community health services • Contact school nurse regarding actions to take during vaso-occlusive crisis **RATIONALE:** *Knowledge of dangerous situations, discussions of how to avoid and manage them reduce risk of serious injury.*
10 Anxiety *r.t. unfamiliarity with cause, treatment, complications, lifestyle disruptions*	• Family/child describe the cause, course and chronic nature of sickle cell anemia	• Assess family/child readiness to learn; when ready, educate regarding - activities when not in crisis - events that precipitate crisis - symptoms of crisis - fluid and nutrition management - actions to take in the event of a crisis - wearing medical ID bracelet
	• Parents express feelings about hereditary disease transmission	• Provide genetic counseling for parents, adolescent child
	• Family/child describe precipitating factors of pain and vaso-occlusive crisis; take appropriate actions to minimize pain and crises	• Discuss factors that precipitate pain and vaso-occlusive crisis • Identify actions to minimize pain and crisis

MEDICAL

NURSING DIAGNOSES	OUTCOME CRITERIA	INTERVENTIONS
	• Parent/child discuss pathophysiology of disease process, rationale for treatment	• Explain disease pathophysiology, treatments, medications, prognosis; explain need for prophylactic penicillin for splenectomized child
	• Parent/child discuss s/s of impending crisis: fever, pain, lethargy, pallor, anorexia, vomiting, headaches, cyanosis, urinary frequency	• Describe, provide list of reportable s/s
	• Wears medical ID band; identifies reasons for regular follow-up care • Accepts reality that there is some chance that surgery may eventually be necessary	• Assist in obtaining medical ID bracelet, band; refer to home care coordinator, community health nurse, hematologist, sickle cell clinic as indicated

RATIONALE: *Increased family knowledge enables them to participate in the decision-making for planning of care and minimizing crises. A knowledgeable family is likely to safely manage home care.*

OTHER LESS COMMON NURSING DIAGNOSES: *Hyperthermia; Altered Nutrition: Less than body requirements; Fear; Altered Growth and Development; Self-Care Deficit*

ESSENTIAL DISCHARGE CRITERIA

- Exhibits no s/s of vaso-occlusive crisis
- Displays adequate hydration
- Maintains pain control with oral medication
- Parents demonstrate required care techniques

- Parent/child identify community sources for emergency and routine care
- Parent/child identify community resources for support as needed

SYSTEMIC LUPUS ERYTHEMATOSUS

NURSING DIAGNOSES	OUTCOME CRITERIA	INTERVENTIONS
1 Activity Intolerance *r.t. weakness, aching, malaise*	• Increases activity to maintain prior energy level - performs ADL - exercises regularly - attends school/work - identifies factors that aggravate activity intolerance	• Encourage a balance of exercise and rest • Pace activity • Allow time to finish a task • Allow for short breaks • Provide physical therapy as ordered **RATIONALE:** *Fatigue and stress contribute to recurrence of symptoms.*
2 Fatigue *r.t. chronic inflammation*	• Shares feelings regarding fatigue's effects on daily life • Establishes priorities for activities • Knows how to decrease workload on the system	• Discuss impact of fatigue on ADLs • Encourage adequate rest periods • Organize daily tasks • Moderate activity • Teach family/friends about patient's need for rest • Help develop a diet plan to reduce weight and conserve energy **RATIONALE:** *Fatigue is one factor contributing to reoccurrence of symptoms.*
3 Chronic Pain *r.t. fibroid deposition in connective tissue* *(Refer to "Pain Management" care plan)*	• Communicates reduced pain - increases use of hands and feet - exhibits increased energy level - provides subjective data regarding pain relief	• Assess pain level on children's pain scale - observe nonverbal cues • Administer analgesics as ordered; assess for effectiveness • Teach patient's family about need for regular medication **RATIONALE:** *Proper use of medication can prevent inflammatory symptoms leading to pain.*

MEDICAL

NURSING DIAGNOSES	OUTCOME CRITERIA	INTERVENTIONS
4 Anxiety *r.t. change in body image*	• Has positive, healthy self-image - participates in activities per age - develops positive relationships	• Support positive behaviors - allow outlet for feelings - refer to support groups for adolescents (SLE societies) • Increase social contacts
		RATIONALE: *Adolescents relate closely to peers. Social contact is important to normal growth and development.*
5 Impaired Skin Integrity *r.t. inflammation of connective tissue, altered circulation, medications, immobility*	• Skin is clear, intact - skin lesions clearing - no localized redness, purulent drainage - hand, feet are warm	• Monitor, protect skin integrity - inspect skin q8h: note size, character, location of rash, lesions, ulcerations - keep lesions clean, dry; apply ordered topical ointments; assess effects - use eggcrate, sheepskin; warmth to extremities - protect from fluorescent, sunlight
		RATIONALE: *Prolonged exposure to sunlight or an infection can exacerbate well-controlled SLE.*
6 Altered Thought Processes *r.t. neurologic involvement*	• Is neurologically stable: no seizures, ptosis, nystagmus, diplopia	• Assess LOC q4h
	• Is alert, oriented	• Orient to time, place, person, activity prn; provide familiar objects
	• Sleeps, naps WNL for age	• Maintain calm, quiet environment during rest periods
	• Sustains no seizure-related injuries	• Initiate seizure precautions; keep side rails up
		RATIONALE: *Confusion is one of the major symptoms which may signal an exacerbation of well-controlled SLE.*

NURSING DIAGNOSES	OUTCOME CRITERIA	INTERVENTIONS
7 Fluid Volume Excess *r.t. steroids*	• Body weight is stable, WNL	• Weigh daily
	• Shows BP WNL	• Monitor BP q4-8h
	• Maintains balanced I&O	• Maintain strict I&O
	• Urine shows no hematuria, proteinuria; sp. gr. WNL	• Dipstick all urine; monitor sp. gr. q4-8h
	• BUN, creatinine WNL	• Monitor lab values qd
	• Has no edema	• Inspect extremities for edema q8h; elevate extremities • Administer ordered diuretics, steroids, antihypertensives
		RATIONALE: *Problems associated with steroids (i.e., weight gain due to Na and fluid retention, and increased appetite) require vigilant assessment.*
8 Decreased Cardiac Output *r.t. inflammation of cardiac tissue*	• Shows ECG, VS stable, WNL	• Monitor VS, ECG q4h, prn; report arrhythmias
	• Has normal peripheral pulses; capillary refill WNL	• Assess peripheral pulses, capillary refill q4-8h
	• Exhibits no cyanosis, pallor, restlessness	• Assess skin color and warmth, restlessness q4h
	• Experiences no dyspnea, orthopnea, irregular respirations	• Assess respiratory status q4h; keep O_2 at bedside; report respiratory distress
		RATIONALE: *Decreased cardiac output can lead to dyspnea, arrhythmias, or cyanosis.*

MEDICAL

SYSTEMIC LUPUS ERYTHEMATOSUS

NURSING DIAGNOSES	OUTCOME CRITERIA	INTERVENTIONS
9 Diversional Activity Deficit *r.t. photosensitivity*	• Parent/child discuss ways to limit sun exposure	• Explain how to limit exposure to sun 　- suggest clothing, PABA sunscreen to face, large-brimmed hat 　- suggest staying indoors between 10 a.m. and 4 p.m. 　- encourage performance of "normal" tasks, driving, shopping **RATIONALE:** *Ultraviolet rays aggravate skin lesions.*
10 Knowledge Deficit *r.t. diagnosis, pathophysiology, medications, care techniques*	• Parent/child discuss pathophysiology of disease process, rationale for treatment, prognosis; express feelings, ask appropriate questions	• Allow specific times, private place to teach 　- pathophysiology, treatment, complications, prognosis 　- physical limitations
	• Parents list medication effects, side effects, dosages	• Explain medications: effects, side effects • Give information about 　- aspirin Rx 　- steroid Rx 　- antimalarial Rx • Explain lowered resistance to sun exposure • Explain risk of infection • Explain need to monitor CBC
	• Parent/child list reportable s/s: extremes of weight, skin ulcerations, fever, bleeding, cyanosis, dyspnea, altered LOC	• Describe complications, reportable s/s
	• Parent/child participate in care activities; demonstrate required home care techniques	• Demonstrate required care techniques; explain journal-keeping, diet, rest
	• Parent/child discuss, experiment with esthetic enhancements	• Provide suggestions for body image changes: make-up, scarves, wigs, clothing
	• Parent/child involved with counselor, community health nurse, National SLE Foundation as indicated	• Refer to counselor, social worker, community health nurse as indicated; verify possession of follow-up appointments **RATIONALE:** *Patients have the need and responsibility to be aware of how SLE affects their bodies, including the effects of medications and treatments.*

OTHER LESS COMMON NURSING DIAGNOSES: Ineffective Individual Coping; Altered Family Processes; Altered Tissue Perfusion (renal)

ESSENTIAL DISCHARGE CRITERIA

- Afebrile, no s/s of infection
- Shows skin lesions clearing, absent
- Reports/displays reasonable comfort; sleeps, naps WNL for age

- Parents demonstrate required care techniques and list reportable s/s
- Parent/child express confidence in ability to manage at home; identify required support success

TUBERCULOSIS

NURSING DIAGNOSES	OUTCOME CRITERIA	INTERVENTIONS

1 Ineffective Airway Clearance
 	
r.t. bacterial lung infection
	• Maintains a clear airway
	  - shows RR WNL
	  - clear and equal breath sounds bilaterally
	  - no persistent cough, aching pain or tightness in the chest, stridor
	  - temperature WNL
	  - improving chest x-ray, with absence of atelectasis and pleural effusion
		• Assess and record the following q4h and prn
		  - RR and temperature
		  - breath sounds
		  - any s/s of ineffective airway clearance
		
		• Administer bacteriocidal anti-tuberculosis agents (e.g., isoniazid, rifampin, streptomycin) on schedule
		
		• Assess and record effectiveness of any medication side effects (GI discomfort, hypersensitivity reactions, neurologic complications)
		
		• Administer antipyretics if indicated; record effectiveness
		
		• Administer O_2 per orders
		  - record percent of O_2 and route of delivery
		  - assess and record effectiveness
		
		• Provide chest physiotherapy per orders; record effects
		
		• Suction gently if unable to clear airway
		
		• Elevate HOB at 30° angle (may use infant seat if infant can support head in midline position)
		
		• Review results of chest x-ray

	• Takes adequate fluids to help liquify secretions	• Monitor I&O • Encourage fluid intake; regulate IV fluids per orders
	• Demonstrates understanding of secretion containment	• Instruct child to spit out secretions in a tissue and dispose in waste container; adhere to CDC guidelines and/or institutional policy for precaution/isolation techniques
		RATIONALE: *Providing anti-tuberculosis agents combined with secretive liquification, reclining, and positioning fosters healing and drainage of potentially obstructive secretions.*

NURSING DIAGNOSES	OUTCOME CRITERIA	INTERVENTIONS
2 High Risk for Infection (transmission) *r.t. contagious nature of infection*	• Remains in isolation until free of active virus	• Maintain universal precautions • Maintain strict isolation procedures per agency protocol, CDC precautions • Enforce strict hand-washing procedures • Use disposable utensils
		RATIONALE: *Isolation precautions reduce chance of transmission.*

3 Knowledge Deficit
 	
r.t. unfamiliarity with communicability of tuberculosis, cultural and language differences, guilt associated with child's acquiring tuberculosis
	• Parent/child have adequate knowledge concerning the child's illness and care
	  - correctly state information regarding tuberculosis and the child's care (communicability, need to identify the source of the child's illness, testing for other family members, home care, medication administration, compliance with treatment, future testing of a child)
	  - correctly demonstrate skills (medication administration, hygiene)
	  - relate appropriate information to care providers
		• Listen to parents' concerns and fears
		• Assess parents' knowledge and understanding of illness
		• Assess parents' knowledge of and participation in care regarding
		  - hygiene
		  - nutrition
		  - activity level
		  - medication administration
		  - isolation from susceptible others
		• Assist and observe parents in performing care techniques; clarify misconceptions
		• Assign one nurse as primary resource to parents; obtain interpreter as required

	• Parents have follow-up appointments and know community resources	• Verify parents' knowledge of and realistic ability to manage follow-up care appointments • Refer to community support services to assist with compliance
		RATIONALE: *Tuberculosis requires a long recovery period during which the parents will be responsible for care. Knowledgeable, competent parents who know how and when to seek help will be more successful.*

MEDICAL

237

> ### OTHER LESS COMMON NURSING DIAGNOSES:
> *Activity Intolerance; Altered Nutrition: Less than body requirements; Noncompliance*

ESSENTIAL DISCHARGE CRITERIA

- Takes anti-tuberculosis medications without side effects
- Parent/child demonstrate compliance with CDC precautions and/or isolation
- Parents demonstrate safe, effective care techniques
- Parents have referrals to community resources and follow-up appointments with physician

NURSING DIAGNOSES	OUTCOME CRITERIA	INTERVENTIONS
1 Diarrhea *r.t. colon inflammation*	• Achieves, maintains balanced I&O	• Maintain strict I&O; assess q8h
	• Shows decreasing frequency of stools	• Note status of diarrhea - frequency, amount, consistency, color - precipitating factors
	• Has soft, formed stools	• Provide smooth, soft, bland diet as ordered
	• Verbalizes, displays decreased cramping, pain	• Administer ordered corticosteroids, bowel sedatives; assess effects, side effects
		RATIONALE: *Adequate hydration, bland diet, and antiflammatory medications reduce bowel hypermotility.*
2 High Risk for Fluid Volume Deficit *r.t. diarrhea*	• Achieves, maintains balanced I&O	• Monitor I&O
	• Shows stable body weight, WNL	• Weigh daily
	• Displays good skin turgor, moist mucous membranes	• Inspect skin, mucous membranes q4-8h
	• Shows serum electrolytes, Hct, Hb, Ca, BUN WNL	• Monitor electrolytes, Hct, Hb, Ca, BUN
	• Shows urinary sp. gr. WNL	• Assess urinary sp. gr. as ordered
	• Exhibits no s/s of muscular atony, lethargy, confusion	• Observe for s/s of Na, K, Ca, prothrombin depletion q4-8h
		RATIONALE: *Monitoring hydration and providing fluids counteract fluid loss associated with diarrhea.*

MEDICAL

NURSING DIAGNOSES	OUTCOME CRITERIA	INTERVENTIONS

3 High Risk for Impaired Skin Integrity
 	
 r.t. diarrheal excoriation
	• Displays clear, intact skin
	 • Shows no localized redness, purulent drainage
		• Protect perianal skin
		   - clean perineum after each stool
		   - provide sitz baths; expose to air; apply protective creams, ointments
		
		 RATIONALE: *Cleansing and protection reduce risk of excoriation. Exposure to air dries area, reducing bacterial growth.*

4 Pain (chronic) *r.t. edema and irritability of colon* *(Refer to "Pain Management" care plan)*	• Verbalizes reduction in or absence of pain	• Assess for abdominal cramping • Administer analgesic and anticholinergic as ordered • Provide bed rest and reduce stimuli **RATIONALE:** *These measures reduce pain and promote rest to help decrease edema and irritability of the colon.*
5 High Risk for Altered Nutrition: Less than body requirements *r.t. inability to absorb nutrients*	• Demonstrates behaviors and lifestyle changes that regain and/or maintain appropriate weight	• Provide and encourage a high-protein, high-calorie, high-vitamin diet • Teach how to reduce intake of milk and milk products **RATIONALE:** *Providing a proper diet helps patient to maintain appropriate body weight.*
6 Family Coping: Potential for growth *r.t. chronicity of disease*	• Parent/child express feelings • Child makes positive self-reports, asserts self	• Allow time for discussion of feelings, sense of self
	• Child initiates interactions with staff, peers	• Facilitate opportunities for positive interactions with staff, peers
	• Child takes normal periods of rest	• Encourage frequent rest periods
	• Parent/child identify coping difficulties; identify at least one new coping skill	• Assist family to identify one needed coping skill; offer positive feedback for positive coping behaviors

NURSING DIAGNOSES	OUTCOME CRITERIA	INTERVENTIONS
	• Family, child involved with counseling as indicated	• Refer to counseling as indicated
		RATIONALE: *Fostering feedback and problem-solving reinforces long-term coping skills.*
7 Knowledge Deficit *r.t. complex management of care, prevention of exacerbations*	• Parent/child discuss physiology of disease process, rationale for treatment	• Explain pathophysiology of disease; discuss treatment rationale
	• Parent/child discuss, demonstrate required care techniques	• Demonstrate required care techniques
	• Parent/child describe s/s of exacerbation: frequent, liquid stools; oliguria; pain, cramping; lethargy	• Provide list of reportable s/s of exacerbation, infection
	• Parent/child discuss medications: effects, side effects, dosages	• Explain medications: effects, side effects, dosages, times delivered
	• Parent/child select required foods from list	• Include dietitian in nutrition teaching
	• Family possesses follow-up appointment	• Refer to community health nurse, other resources as indicated; verify possession of follow-up appointment
		RATIONALE: *Knowledgeable, competent parents are likely to successfully manage the child's long-term care.*

MEDICAL

> **OTHER LESS COMMON NURSING DIAGNOSES:** *Anxiety; High Risk for Fluid Volume Deficit;*
> *High Risk for Injury (bowel perforation)*

ESSENTIAL DISCHARGE CRITERIA

- Reports that pain is under control

- Demonstrates ability to reduce stimuli and to rest when needed

- Stooling frequency and consistency are within acceptable limits

- Parent/child demonstrate accurate knowledge of appropriate diet

- Parent/child verbalize plan for home care and possess follow-up appointments.

NURSING DIAGNOSES	OUTCOME CRITERIA	INTERVENTIONS

1 Fluid Volume Deficit
 	
r.t. active fluid loss, surgical removal of kidney
	• Maintains fluid volume at a functional level
	  - stable VS
	  - individually adequate urinary output with normal sp. gr.
	  - moist mucous membranes
	  - good skin turgor
	  - capillary refill < 3 sec
	  - normal lab results
		• Assess, document vital signs q2-4h
		• Maintain adequate I&O q shift
		• Test urinary sp. gr. as ordered
		• Assess physical signs: concentrated urine, dry mucous membranes, delayed capillary refill, poor skin turgor, confusion
		• Review laboratory data: Hb, Hct, electrolytes, total protein and albumin, BUN, creatinine
		
		RATIONALE: *Monitoring these signs will allow early detection and correction of imbalances.*

2 Knowledge Deficit
 	
r.t. new diagnosis of Wilms' Tumor
 	
(Refer to "Cancer" care plan)
 	
(Refer to "Chemotherapy" care plan)
 	
(Refer to "Radiation Therapy" care plan)
	• Family/child demonstrate knowledge and competence
	  - participate in learning process
	  - verbalize understanding of disease process and treatment
	  - perform necessary procedures correctly and explain reasons for the actions
	  - initiate necessary lifestyle changes
	  - participate in treatment regimen
		• Determine level of knowledge, including anticipatory needs
		• Provide chemotherapy drug cards and explain side effects and management
		• Provide information regarding radiation therapy
		  - facilitate child and family touring radiation therapy department before discharge
		• Reinforce information provided by doctors and radiation therapy staff
		• Provide written and verbal information regarding Wilm's tumor
		• Document teaching done and patient/family's assimilation of information
		
		RATIONALE: *Understanding of the disease, treatment, and potential outcomes leads to better maintenance of the child's health at home.*

MEDICAL

OTHER LESS COMMON NURSING DIAGNOSES:
Anxiety; Pain; Altered Family Processes; High Risk for Injury

ESSENTIAL DISCHARGE CRITERIA

- Lab values are within acceptable limits
- Is afebrile
- Exhibits no signs of infection

- Family/child verbalize plan for home care, compliance with follow-up care, and list reportable s/s

SURGICAL NURSING

CONTENTS

SURGICAL

APPENDECTOMY

NURSING DIAGNOSES	OUTCOME CRITERIA	INTERVENTIONS

See "Preoperative" and "Postoperative" care plans

1 Pain

r.t. surgical incision

- Displays comfort behavior
  - relaxed body posture, facial expression
  - does not moan or guard incision
  - naps, sleeps qs
  - ambulates on schedule without undue resistance

- Assess, control pain q2-3h
- Administer ordered analgesics; assess relief
- Provide distraction, diversion, back rubs, holding
- Provide uninterrupted nap, sleep periods
- Involve parents in active partnership to plan and provide comfort and diversion

RATIONALE: *Timely pain control reduces episodic pain and stress. Parents know accustomed methods for diverting and comforting the child.*

---

2 High Risk for Infection

r.t. surgical incision

- Remains afebrile

- Monitor VS q4h

- Displays soft, undistended abdomen; presents no guarding

- Examine abdomen for rigidity, tenderness q4-8h
- Measure abdominal girth if indicated

- Exhibits incision free of redness, drainage; edges are approximated

- Inspect wound q2-4h
- Reinforce packing if wound is open
- Change dressing when saturated
- Teach parents how to inspect, care for incision

RATIONALE: *Early detection and treatment of s/s of incisional infection reduce risk of peritonitis.*

---

3 Constipation

r.t. anesthesia, abdominal pain

- Has normal bowel sounds

- Assess bowel sounds q4h

- Shows no abdominal distention

- Inspect abdomen
- Measure abdominal girth if indicated

NURSING DIAGNOSES	OUTCOME CRITERIA	INTERVENTIONS
	• Passes soft, formed stool q1-2 days	• Encourage mobility • Advance diet as tolerated; report nausea, vomiting
		RATIONALE: *Early detection and management of diminished bowel activity reduce the possibility of constipation.*
4 Knowledge Deficit *r.t. inexperience with postoperative course*	• Parents discuss expected course of recovery, ask appropriate questions	• Explain expected course of convalescence; allow time for parents to ask questions, express concerns
	• Parents demonstrate required wound care, if any	• Demonstrate any required wound care with aseptic technique
	• Parents verbalize knowledge of s/s of distension, fever, pain	• Provide list of s/s of complications that should be reported to physician
	• Parents verbalize knowledge of follow-up appointments	• Verify knowledge of follow-up appointments
		RATIONALE: *When parents can discuss and ask questions and also demonstrate required skills, there is increased likelihood of a safe, uncomplicated recovery.*

SURGICAL

OTHER LESS COMMON NURSING DIAGNOSES: Altered Body Image; Altered Nutrition: Less than body requirements; Fluid Volume Deficit

---

ESSENTIAL DISCHARGE CRITERIA

• Is afebrile

• Has no abdominal distention, rigidity; passes stool

• Takes 90% of recommended nutrition

• At least one parent demonstrates any required wound care

• Parents list reportable s/s and possess follow-up appointment

BURNS AND GRAFTS

NURSING DIAGNOSES	OUTCOME CRITERIA	INTERVENTIONS

See "Preoperative" and "Postoperative" care plans

1 Fluid Volume Deficit

r.t. shift of intravascular fluids to interstitial spaces; fluid loss from evaporation at burn site

- Shows adequate fluid volume and electrolyte balance
  - VS, BP WNL
  - stable weight
  - adequate urinary output
  - electrolytes WNL
  - afebrile
  - urinary sp. gr. WNL
  - moist mucous membranes

- Monitor VS q15min until stable, then q1-2h
- Monitor I&O
- Weigh patient daily at same time
- Monitor serum electrolytes
- Monitor urinary sp. gr. q2h
- Observe for signs of circulatory overload (dyspnea, rales, neck distension, including CVP)
- Administer replacement K therapy for hypokalemia as ordered
- Administer IV therapy as ordered

RATIONALE: *Prevent further fluid loss and minimize complications.*

2 Pain

r.t. exposed nerve endings and edema due to burn injury

(Refer to "Pain" care plan)

- Verbalizes/displays reasonable comfort

- Assess and record HR, BP, and respirations
- Assess the level of discomfort using a 0-10-point self-rating scale to obtain an objective measure

- Achieves, maintains sustained comfort

- Perform pharmacological interventions as ordered by the physician
  - medicate with maximal dose to break pain cycle as long as LOC, HR, BP are stable
  - instruct to ask for pain medication when pain is beginning and not to wait until pain is intolerable
  - re-evaluate pain medication 5 min after IV; 20 min after IM; monitor VS and behavior and ask patient to rate pain using the scale
  - explain that if pain relief is inadequate with the present medication, alternatives will be tried

NURSING DIAGNOSES	OUTCOME CRITERIA	INTERVENTIONS
	• Reports reasonable comfort during dressing changes, physical therapy	• Perform rehabilitation exercises, physical therapy, or wound dressing changes shortly before peak of drug effects
	• Actively participates in nonpharmacologic pain control techniques	• Explain other treatments such as relaxation techniques, diversion, music therapy, or imagery to decrease pain • Position patient for comfort
	• Maintains body temperature WNL; no episodes of chilling, shivering	• Maintain a warm environment at approximately 24.4-28°C (76-82°F) to ensure warmth and comfort; monitor patient's temperature q2h • Consider referral for hydrotherapy
		RATIONALE: *Pain causes symptoms of increased BP, HR, and respirations, as well as pupillary dilation, diaphoresis, pallor, grimacing, clenching fists, and apprehension. Scheduling of analgesia so that it is at its peak effect at the time of activity or dressing changes is necessary to prevent pain.*
3 Impaired Skin Integrity *r.t. partial thickness or full thickness burn*	• Experiences no further skin impairment	• Assess the skin integrity q4h during acute phase and q8h thereafter; record and report any color changes in the skin, mucous membranes, nail beds • Turn q2h, or more often if bony prominences remain erythematous for more than 15 min after pressure is relieved (erythema unresolved within 15 min indicates tissue ischemia) • Prevent skin shear and friction - allow feet to rest against footboard when HOB elevated - do not elevated HOB higher than 30° (to decrease sliding) - provide heel and elbow protectors - use lift sheet to reposition • Apply tape without tension to prevent blistering

SURGICAL

NURSING DIAGNOSES	OUTCOME CRITERIA	INTERVENTIONS
		• Remove tape by peeling away while stabilizing skin, or use gauze or Montgomery straps to secure dressings
		• Avoid all unnecessary use of adhesive on skin
		• Keep skin as clean and dry as possible at all times
		• Change dressings using sterile technique

RATIONALE: *These measures help to prevent further skin breakdown, prevent pressure and trauma to injured tissue.*

NURSING DIAGNOSES	OUTCOME CRITERIA	INTERVENTIONS
4 **Altered Tissue Perfusion (renal, cardio-pulmonary, gastrointestinal and peripheral)** *r.t. hypovolemia, peripheral edema*	• Maintains adequate systemic tissue perfusion - VS, BP WNL - unlabored respirations - urinary output > 30 mL/h - no urinary hematuria or discoloration - skin warm, dry - palpable peripheral pulses	• Assess and report any s/s of decreased tissue perfusion - monitor VS q1-4h; report any significant decrease in BP, HR > 100 bpm, labored respirations - monitor urinary output; report output < 30 mL/h - observe for hematuria (or brownish-red, indicating intravascular hemolysis) - monitor skin color; report cool, pale, mottled, or cyanotic skin in unburned areas - palpate peripheral pulses; report absence or decrease in quality (peripheral pulses should be marked and checked with doppler flow meter qh for 48h post-burn or until edema subsides)
	• Peripheral edema diminishes	• Assess and record presence of edema; if present, attempt to elevate extremity above level of heart
	• Shows decrease in circumference of burned areas	• Measure circumference of burned area to determine if edema is increasing - assist with escharotomy or fasciotomy of circumferential burns
	• Shows no changes in baseline LOC	• Report any changes in LOC, restlessness or confusion

NURSING DIAGNOSES	OUTCOME CRITERIA	INTERVENTIONS
	• Adjusts to position changes without dizziness, fainting	• Change patient's position slowly to allow time for autoregulatory mechanisms to adjust to position change • Maintain adequate fluid replacement • Maintain optimal mobility • Provide adequate nutrition
		RATIONALE: *Measures to optimize fluid, electrolyte, and nutritional balance help to maintain circulation, circulating volume, and promote tissue healing.*

5 Altered Nutrition: Less than body requirements
 	
r.t. increased caloric and protein needs for wound healing and metabolic response
	• Exhibits balanced metabolic state
	  - stable weight
	  - serum electrolytes WNL
	  - progressive wound healing
	  - nutritional intake maintained within 90% of calculated nutritional needs
		• Monitor I&O
		
		• Provide high-protein, high-calorie diet as ordered
		
		• Observe for s/s of dehydration
		
		• Weigh daily
		
		• Encourage PO intake, small frequent feedings
		
		• Administer tube feedings per orders
		
		• Minimize energy requirements
		
		• Anticipate need for TPN; administer as ordered

		RATIONALE: *Adequate nutritional intake promotes wound healing.*

6 Impaired Gas Exchange
 	
r.t. ineffective airway clearance secondary to edema/obstruction, inhalation injury, damaged pulmonary tissue, carbon monoxide poisoning
	• Maintain adequate O_2 exchange
	  - unlabored respirations
	  - SaO_2 WNL
	  - clear bilateral breath sounds
	  - blood gases WNL
		• Observe for signs of respiratory distress (dyspnea, cyanosis in PaO_2 levels, restlessness, confusion)
		
		• Monitor SaO_2 levels
		
		• Monitor ABG levels
		
		• Elevate HOB 30°
		
		• Administer humidified O_2 per order
		
		• Encourage deep breathing, coughing, turning q2h
		
		• Perform endotracheal or nasotracheal suction as needed

SURGICAL

NURSING DIAGNOSES	OUTCOME CRITERIA	INTERVENTIONS
		• Monitor need for ventilatory support
		RATIONALE: *Prevent imbalance between O₂ uptake and CO₂ elimination and minimize complications.*

NURSING DIAGNOSES	OUTCOME CRITERIA	INTERVENTIONS
7 High Risk for Infection *r.t. multiple invasive procedures, tissue destruction, malnutrition*	• Remians free of infection - negative cultures (blood, sputum, urine) - afebrile - WBC WNL - VS WNL	• Monitor temperature q1-2h; report elevation • Use universal precautions • Maintain hand-washing to minimize cross-contamination • Use strict aseptic technique (gowns, gloves, mask) when performing invasive procedures • Prevent patient exposure to infected visitors/staff • Obtain cultures as ordered; report abnormalities • Monitor CBC and WBC • Discontinue invasive lines as soon as possible • Observe body fluids for changes in color, odor, or consistency • Administer systemic antibiotics • Provide reverse isolation if indicated
		RATIONALE: *Frequent monitoring and prompt management minimize any present infection and prevent future microbial transmission.*

> **OTHER LESS COMMON NURSING DIAGNOSES:** *Impaired Physical Mobility; Altered Nutrition: Less than body requirements; Body Image Disturbance; Ineffective Individual Coping; Knowledge Deficit; Hypothermia; Pain; Fluid Volume Excess; High Risk for Disuse Syndrome*

ESSENTIAL DISCHARGE CRITERIA

- Maintains physiological homeostasis
- Shows blood lab values WNL
- Burn area is healing and free of infection

- Patient/family verbalize/demonstrate understanding of burn healing and therapeutic regimen including wound care
- Patient/family recognize complications; identify when to notify physician

CARDIAC SURGERY

See "Preoperative" and "Postoperative" care plans

1 Anxiety

r.t. surgical procedure, hospitalization

- Parents/child display minimal anxiety; show appropriate coping mechanisms

- Encourage child/parent to verbalize questions or concerns
- Provide instruction related to hospital routine/procedures and illness; provide appropriate pre- and postoperative teaching
- Suggest parents provide favorite toy and pictures of sibling/pets; encourage parental participation in child's care
- Refer to Child Life specialists

RATIONALE: *Knowledge of what to expect, participation in care, and expression of concerns reduce anxiety.*

2 Decreased Cardiac Output

r.t. surgical procedure, dysrhythmias, fluid imbalance

- Manifests adequate cardiac output
  - VS WNL
  - palpable pulses in all extremities
  - extremities warm to touch
  - capillary refill WNL
  - stable respiratory status
  - SaO_2 WNL
  - urine output at least 1 mL/kg/h

- Monitor VS frequently and report changes/abnormalities to physician
- Assess tissue perfusion q15min until stable, then qh x 24h
  - capillary refill
  - quality of pulses
  - urinary output (> 1 mL/kg/h)
- Provide continuous cardio-respiratory monitoring
- Monitor for signs of dysrhythmia
- Assess for cardiac complications
  - bradycardia
  - diminished heart sounds
  - hypotension

- Displays no periorbital or dependent edema
- Lungs are clear
- Shows no gain or fluctuating weight
- Displays no undue restlessness

- Monitor for cardiac/circulatory overload
  - fluid retention/edema
  - respiratory distress
  - weight gain
  - restlessness

NURSING DIAGNOSES	OUTCOME CRITERIA	INTERVENTIONS

	• Chest tube drainage is within acceptable limits for color, amount	• Monitor chest tube drainage
		  - volume, consistency
		  - notify physician if output is equal to or greater than 3-5 mL/kg/h for an hour

		RATIONALE: *Frequent monitoring of cardiac output prompts early detection and management of significant variations.*

3 Ineffective Breathing Pattern
r.t. chest incision
	• Displays effective breathing patterns
	  - RR, depth, quality WNL
	  - no retractions or nasal flaring
	  - bilateral breath sounds clear
	  - no cyanosis present
	  - O_2 sats WNL
		• Monitor respiratory status q1-2h
		  - rate and depth
		  - quality of breath sounds
		• Assess skin color and mucous membranes
		• Monitor ABGs and SaO_2
		• Monitor chest tube drainage consistency and volume
		• Insure that chest tube water seal and/or suction is set properly
		  - check for air leaks
		  - maintain patency; check tubing for obstructions
		• Maintain ordered ventilatory support (if applicable)
		• Assist to turn, cough, and deep breathe q2h
		• Encourage child to engage in play activities to facilitate lung expansion
		  - blowing bubbles/windmills
		  - pediatric incentive spirometer equipment

		RATIONALE: *Frequent monitoring and implementation of vigorous preventative nursing measures counteract the splinting effect of the incision upon the chest.*

SURGICAL

NURSING DIAGNOSES	OUTCOME CRITERIA	INTERVENTIONS
4 Fluid Volume Deficit *r.t. perioperative fluid loss*	• Displays adequate fluid volume - electrolytes WNL, including BUN, creatinine - urine output at least 1 mL/kg/h - capillary refill < 3 sec - peripheral pulses WNL	• Monitor lab values daily: electrolytes, BUN, and creatinine • Monitor I&O • Monitor capillary refill time • Monitor chest tube output as ordered • Monitor for circulatory overload q15min/h x 1-2d: orthopnea, restlessness, rales, edema, elevated BP
	• Displays moist mucous membranes, good skin turgor, normal fontanel tension (infants)	• Monitor hydration status
	• Remains alert, oriented	• Monitor LOC • Monitor for signs of cardiac arrhythmia
		RATIONALE: *Frequent monitoring of hydration results in early detection of dehydration and produces prompt medical and nursing interventions.*
5 High Risk for Infection *r.t. surgical incision*	• Exhibits no signs of infection - afebrile - no redness, swelling, abnormal drainage - WBC WNL - no pericardial effusion - blood cultures negative	• Monitor and record temperature and report abnormalities to the physician • Assess wound, chest tube, and IV sites for redness, swelling or drainage • Maintain aseptic techniques during all invasive procedures (dressing changes, IV site care) • Change dressings as ordered and prn
		RATIONALE: *Vigilance for signs of infection produces prompt treatment when needed.*

NURSING DIAGNOSES	OUTCOME CRITERIA	INTERVENTIONS
6 Pain *r.t. surgical procedure*	• Displays minimal discomfort/pain - naps, rests periodically - VS WNL - plays without distress	• Assess level of pain regularly • Check VS as indicated • Administer analgesic as ordered; assess effectiveness • Reposition patient comfortably q2h • Encourage sitting and ambulation tid • Engage in diversional activities with child when pain medication is not applicable (blowing bubbles, playing a game, coloring a book, playing video games) **RATIONALE:** *A consistent regimen of pharmacologic and nonpharmacologic techniques produces sustained comfort.*
7 Altered Nutrition: Less than body requirements *r.t. post-op discomfort*	• Displays evidence of adequate nutrition - good/elastic skin turgor - moist mucous membranes - capillary refill < 3 sec - skin free of breakdown - stable weight	• Enforce strict I&O • Administer IV fluids as ordered • Monitor IV site for patency • Encourage PO intake, especially foods high in protein to promote healing • Offer favorite food and foods appropriate for age - toddlers: finger foods (fish sticks, drum sticks, green beans) - school age and adolescents: pizza, hot dogs, baked potatoes **RATIONALE:** *Well-nourished body cells are required to support the healing needed for a large area of surgical invasion.*
8 High Risk for Impaired Skin Integrity *r.t. decreased mobility and pain, altered perfusion*	• Displays clear, intact skin	• Inspect skin q shift • Turn q2h while on bed rest • Encourage sitting and ambulation tid • Encourage out-of-bed play - play room activities - playground - teen room

SURGICAL

257

NURSING DIAGNOSES	OUTCOME CRITERIA	INTERVENTIONS
		• Rotate ECG pads per unit standard
		RATIONALE: *Vigorous attention to skin protection through positional change is required to counteract the immobilizing effects of major surgery, pain, chest tubes, and IV tubes.*
9 Knowledge Deficit *r.t. potential complications, care techniques at home*	• Parents/child discuss surgical physiology, ask appropriate questions	• Explain surgical physiology, expected course of convalescence, child's dependency/independency needs
	• Parents/child identify signs of complications: respiratory distress, edema, fever, pain	• Review reportable s/s; provide emergency phone numbers
	• Parents/child identify permitted, restricted activities	• Discuss child's activity/rest regimen
	• Parents/child discuss medications: effects, side effects, dosages	• Explain medications: effects, side effects, dosages
	• Parents/child perform required care techniques	• Demonstrate required care
	• Parents possess follow-up appointments	• Refer to community agencies as indicated; verify knowledge of follow-up care, supervision
		RATIONALE: *Knowledgeable, competent parents are likely to provide for a safe, uneventful recovery.*

OTHER LESS COMMON NURSING DIAGNOSES: *Altered Growth and Development*

ESSENTIAL DISCHARGE CRITERIA

• Exhibits adequate cardiac output

• Exhibits no edema or signs of infection

• Surgical incision intact

• Displays effective breathing pattern

• Demonstrates adequate fluid and nutritional intake

• Parents/child perform required care

• Parents/child verbalize understanding of the importance of follow-up care; possess follow-up appointments

CLEFT LIP AND CLEFT PALATE REPAIR

NURSING DIAGNOSES	OUTCOME CRITERIA	INTERVENTIONS

See "Preoperative" and "Postoperative" care plans

1 Ineffective Airway Clearance

r.t. effects of anesthesia, postoperative edema, mucus production

- Is free of respiratory complications
  - clear lung sounds
  - normal RR, depth, effort

- Assess respiratory status q2h
  - breath sounds
  - nasal flaring
  - retraction
  - RR
  - grunting
  - color (cyanosis)

- Suction as indicated with attention to suture line

- Reposition infant q2h

RATIONALE: *Repositioning and monitoring respiratory status allow for maintaining a clear airway.*

---

2 High Risk for Infection

r.t. trauma of suture line associated with child sucking hands or other damage to suture line

- Is afebrile

- Monitor temperature q2-4h

- Displays clean, clear incision line with intact sutures

- Cleanse suture line with sterile swabs; use half-strength H_2O_2 to remove crusts; apply prescribed ointment

- Assess suture line for infection, separation after each feeding

- Maintains correctly placed restraints

- Use elbow restraint, jacket or straight restraint; remove q2h for skin care (more often when held)

- Parents demonstrate suture care and application of restraints

- Teach parents to clean, inspect sutures, apply restraints, hold properly, minimize crying

RATIONALE: *The chance of infection is reduced when sutures remain intact. Restraint of child's hands and holding and cuddling reduce the chance of the infant's hands reaching the mouth.*

SURGICAL

NURSING DIAGNOSES	OUTCOME CRITERIA	INTERVENTIONS
3 Altered Nutrition: Less than body requirements *r.t. new feeding technique, postoperative dietary changes*	• Maintains adequate nutritional status - maintains prehospitalization weight or gains weight	• Use effective feeding techniques (cleft palate repair) - use soft, cross-cut nipple or the Breck feeder - place nipple in mouth toward the back of tongue and on the opposite side of the cleft - feed in upright semi-sitting position - burp infant after every 15-30 mL - limit feeding time to 30 min • Use effective feeding techniques (cleft lip repair) - feed through a syringe and soft rubber tubing placed inside cheek • Provide small, frequent feedings • Provide a full-liquid diet postoperatively (up to 3 weeks)
		RATIONALE: *These feeding techniques decrease pressure and prevent damage to the suture line.*
4 Anxiety *r.t. limited opportunity for non-nutritive sucking*	• Shows relaxed body posture most of time	• Reduce frustration; distract - hold in sitting position (not against shoulder) as much as possible - anticipate infant's needs to reduce frustration - provide ROM of arms to reduce frustration - distract with toys, activity
	• Parents demonstrate ability to calm infant; acknowledge fact that infant cannot always be calmed	• Support parents' efforts to soothe infant - demonstrate distraction measures - give positive feedback to parents for positive efforts - assist parents to problem-solve and try alternative methods of calming, distracting, anticipating
		RATIONALE: *A variety of anticipatory distraction and soothing techniques reduce infant's frustration. Parent involvement provides the child with increased hours of soothing and comforting.*

NURSING DIAGNOSES	OUTCOME CRITERIA	INTERVENTIONS

5 Altered Parenting
 	
r.t. stress associated with child's appearance and care needs
	• Family maintains normal lifestyle
	  - incorporate infant's care into family lifestyle
	  - verbalizes feelings about infant's appearance
		• Discuss infant's appearance with family
		  - use simple terms
		  - encourage family visits in hospital
		  - suggest support groups available in the community
		• Provide opportunities for family to interact with infant
		  - positioning
		  - bathing
		  - feeding
		  - bonding
		  - dressing

		RATIONALE: *These nursing measures foster realistic expectations of infant's appearance and help to incorporate infant care into family routines.*

6 Knowledge Deficit
 	
r.t. inexperience with special feeding, holding, restraining, soothing behaviors
	• Parents demonstrate ability to: feed; clean suture line; hold properly; restrain safely; soothe, distract infant	• Educate, support parents in infant care
		  - obtain return demonstrations of all care including feeding methods, innovations
		  - allow parents to practice all care skills in hospital
		  - provide starter supplies: sterile swabs, restraints, feeding bulbs, formula

	• Parents verbalize knowledge of s/s of complications: fever; redness, swelling, separation of suture line; drainage, undue restlessness; decreased I&O	• Describe, provide list of reportable s/s
	• Parents verbalize willingness to consider genetic counseling	• Provide genetic counseling information

	• Parents possess knowledge of follow-up appointments	• Provide home care resources
		  - provide unit phone number for 24h support and problem-solving
		  - make referral for home visit if indicated
		  - verify possession of written follow-up appointments

		RATIONALE: *Knowledgeable, competent parents are likely to manage a safe, uneventful period of healing at home.*

SURGICAL

> **OTHER LESS COMMON NURSING DIAGNOSES:** *Impaired Skin Integrity; Pain*

ESSENTIAL DISCHARGE CRITERIA

- Maintains a clear airway
- Suture line is healing and free of infection
- Takes adequate nutrition to maintain weight gain
- Family demonstrates effective infant feeding techniques
- Parents verbalize plan for follow-up and list s/s reportable to PCP

COLON SURGERY, ADOLESCENT

NURSING DIAGNOSES	OUTCOME CRITERIA	INTERVENTIONS

See "Preoperative" and "Postoperative" care plans

1 Anxiety

r.t. impending surgery, lack of knowledge regarding colostomy care

- Verbalizes fears in relation to surgery

  - Assess level of anxiety
  - Encourage patient to verbalize feelings
  - Provide reassurance and comfort

- Verbalizes expected events following surgery

  - Teach patient what to expect following surgery
  - Provide information regarding colostomy and colostomy care

RATIONALE: *Knowledge of expectations and verbalization of anxiety decrease intensity of the anxiety.*

2 Pain

r.t. surgical procedure

- Identifies source of discomfort

  - Teach and explain cause of discomfort
  - Acknowledge patient's discomfort

- Identifies medication or activity that reduces discomfort
- Alternates periods of activity and rest

  - Discuss pain management options; allow patient to make choices regarding pain relief

- Reports comfort following administration of analgesia

  - Assess discomfort q2h and administer analgesia as prescribed

RATIONALE: *Collaboration with patient provides personal control over the painful experience.*

3 Body Image Disturbance

r.t. colostomy

- Verbalizes acceptance of altered body image

  - Assess and acknowledge patient's current perception of body image
  - Respect patient's need for withdrawal
  - Assist patient in expressing feelings

SURGICAL

NURSING DIAGNOSES	OUTCOME CRITERIA	INTERVENTIONS
	• Looks at, cares for affected body part	• Provide patient information about care of the colostomy
		• Support and praise self-care of colostomy
	• Reviews resources available for colostomy care	• Encourage participation in support groups and follow-up with home health care

RATIONALE: *Acknowledgment and support enhance adaptive behaviors.*

OTHER LESS COMMON NURSING DIAGNOSES: *Impaired Skin Integrity; Altered Nutrition: Less than body requirements; Constipation; Activity Intolerance; High Risk for Infection*

ESSENTIAL DISCHARGE CRITERIA

- Maintains physiologic homeostasis
- Takes prescribed diet
- Verbalizes plan for relief of discomfort by analgesia or activity at home

- Performs total personal care of colostomy and verbalizes understanding of therapeutic regimen
- Recognizes complications and when to notify PCP

FUNDOLPLICATION

NURSING DIAGNOSES	OUTCOME CRITERIA	INTERVENTIONS

See "Preoperative" and "Postoperative" care plans

1 High Risk for Infection

r.t. surgical invasion

- Shows normal VS, BP
- Exhibits < 3 sec capillary refill time

- Assess and monitor for changes in VS, BP, CRT

- Exhibits normal breath sounds

- Assess respiratory status q2-4h; auscultate breath sounds
- Turn patient regularly; assist to cough and to breathe deeply

---

- Displays intact skin around wounds, tube; no redness, swelling, purulent drainage

- Monitor lab studies: cultures WBC; report deviations from normal
- Demonstrate to patient and family appropriate method of handling wounds, tubes, and secretions

---

RATIONALE: *These measures help prevent infection and assist in early identification of complications.*

---

2 Pain

r.t. distention

- Manifests minimal pain; decreased c/o pain

- Assess need for, and provide pain relief measures
- Change position frequently and administer skin care
- Maintain bed rest in position of comfort

- Exhibits normal bowel sounds

- Auscultate bowel sounds
- Assess frequency of bowel movement, need for pharmacologies

---

- Displays no rigidity of abdomen

- Assess for rigidity of abdomen
- Observe for loops of bowel, abdominal discoloration

RATIONALE: *Provide comfort but monitor for a potential bowel obstruction. Analgesia can mask the pain of bowel obstruction.*

SURGICAL

NURSING DIAGNOSES	OUTCOME CRITERIA	INTERVENTIONS
3 Altered Nutrition: Less than body requirements *r.t. dysphagia/gas bloat syndrome*	• Maintains or regains weight	• Weigh daily • Provide feedings as ordered
	• Shows normal serum electrolytes, Hb, Hct, serum albumin	• Monitor lab reports: electrolytes, Hb, Hct, serum albumin
	• Swallows, retains feedings	• Instruct patient and family about need for techniques to facilitate swallowing
	• Maintains normal GI function (normal bowel movements)	• Assess and monitor for changes in bowel function

RATIONALE: *Adequate nutrition is required for growth and healing.*

OTHER LESS COMMON NURSING DIAGNOSES: *Impaired Tissue Integrity; Ineffective Airway Clearance; Ineffective Infant Feeding Pattern*

ESSENTIAL DISCHARGE CRITERIA

- Takes, retains 90% of feedings
- Gains weight
- Incision is healing with no signs of infection

- Parents demonstrate required home care skills and verbalize plan of care
- Parents verbalize plan for follow-up and list complications to report to PCP

GASTROSTOMY

See "Preoperative" and "Postoperative" care plans

1 High Risk for Altered Nutrition: Less than body requirements

r.t. surgical procedure, parents lack of knowledge regarding gastrostomy feeding

• Exhibits normal values for protein and electrolytes	• Monitor lab values
• Retains 90% of feeding	• Monitor for patency of gastrostomy • Check for stomach residuals before each feeding - accommodate residuals per physician order/unit standards • Administer feeding while giving infant/child positive feeding cues (holding, talking, embracing, rocking) • Administer feeding at a rate that minimizes potential for rapid gastric distention • Flush tubing with water or air after each feeding to facilitate patency
• Maintains balanced I&O	• Record all intake • Record all drainage and output
• Shows consistent weight gain	• Weigh daily
• Has active bowel sounds; no distention	• Assess bowel sounds q4h; observe for distention of abdomen
• Shows gastric residual from prior feed within parameters	• Measure residual before feeding; delay if more than ordered parameters • Vent stomach post feedings until clamp routine initiated

RATIONALE: *Monitoring presence of residual food prevents gastric distention and indicates tolerance of feeding.*

SURGICAL

267

NURSING DIAGNOSES	OUTCOME CRITERIA	INTERVENTIONS
2 Impaired Skin Integrity *r.t. surgery, excretions, secretions*	• Remains afebrile	• Monitor VS q4-8h
	• Shows no evidence of redness or inflammation at gastrostomy site	• Cleanse skin around tube q8h and prn with mild soap and water; rinse thoroughly and pat dry • Allow skin around site to be open to air • Use tape bridge of tubing to secure tube to abdomen • Place gastrostomy clamp near proximal end of the tube when tube is not in use, or per physician order
		RATIONALE: *Preventing strain or accidental dislodging of tube eliminates pressure and skin irritation. Clamping the tube prevents regurgitation of food.*
3 Knowledge Deficit *r.t. lack of experience with gastrostomy care, care beyond cognitive abilities*	• Patient/family demonstrate gastrostomy feedings utilizing proper technique	• Allow patient/family to participate in gastrostomy care and feeding • Teach patient and family how to prepare foods in blender and to select a balanced diet • Observe patient/family performing gastrostomy care with immediate feedback and support • Give patient/family written instructions for home use • Obtain dietary consultation for patient/family regarding commonly used enteral feedings and daily fluid requirement
		RATIONALE: *Patient/family will be able to perform procedure successfully if they learn it actively with support of staff.*

NURSING DIAGNOSES	OUTCOME CRITERIA	INTERVENTIONS

4 Anxiety
r.t. lifestyle change
	• Patient/family verbalize an increase in psychological comfort with caring for gastrostomy	• Allow patient/family to verbalize concerns
		• Arrange for visitation of former patients with gastrostomies
		• Reassure and comfort family while procedure is being learned
		  - stay throughout the procedure
		  - speak slowly and calmly in short, direct sentences
		  - convey empathetic understanding

RATIONALE: *Knowledge and competence reduce anxiety. Understanding how others deal with same problem demystifies the future and reduces tension.*

> ***OTHER LESS COMMON NURSING DIAGNOSES:*** Activity Intolerance; Pain

ESSENTIAL DISCHARGE CRITERIA

- Takes and retains 90% of feedings
- Exhibits no inflammation at stoma site
- Patient/family demonstrate proper gastrostomy care and feeding procedures

- Patient/family verbalize knowledge regarding balanced diets for gastrostomy feedings
- Parents verbalize plans for follow-up and list s/s of complications to report to PCP

SURGICAL

HEAD TRAUMA, SURGICAL MANAGEMENT

NURSING DIAGNOSES	OUTCOME CRITERIA	INTERVENTIONS

See "Preoperative" and "Postoperative" care plans

1 Ineffective Breathing Pattern

r.t. anesthesia, increased ICP, neurogenic pulmonary edema, pulmonary contusion

- Demonstrates normal pulmonary function
  - normal RR for age
  - equal and clear breath sounds
  - unlabored respiratory effort
  - ABGs WNL for age

- Monitor VS (rates age-appropriate)
- Monitor and report changes in respiratory effort
  - tachypnea
  - pulmonary congestion
  - color and consistency of secretions
  - auscultate bilateral breath sounds
  - monitor ABGs and pulse oximetry
- Obtain history of child's injury and surgical intervention, length of anesthesia, drug therapy, and pulmonary status
- Manage spontaneous ventilation
  - assess respiratory effort
  - monitor gag reflex and ability to handle secretions (electively intubate should airway protective mechanisms decrease)
- Manage assisted ventilation
  - assess airway patency and effectiveness of ventilatory support
  - monitor pulse oximetry
  - monitor VS
  - maintain PaO_2 and $PaCO_2$ within ordered limits (elevated $PaCO_2$ potentiates increased ICP)
  - protect child from self-extubation (restrain if necessary)
  - hyperventilate with 100% FiO_2 prior to endotracheal suctioning
  - administer sedatives/paralyzing agents as ordered to maximize ventilatory support

RATIONALE: *These measures prevent hypoxia which accentuates the complications of increased ICP.*

NURSING DIAGNOSES	OUTCOME CRITERIA	INTERVENTIONS
2 Altered Tissue Perfusion (systemic) *r.t. hemorrhage, increased ICP, electrolyte imbalance, hypoxemia*	• Shows HR, BP WNL for age	• Assess and monitor VS, BP qh or as indicated
	• Maintains normal systemic perfusion - no deterioration in LOC - urinary output 1-2 mL/kg/h - skin warm with brisk capillary refill - palpable pedal pulses	• Assess CRT and pedal pulses q1-4h • Assess and monitor neurologic status q2-4h • Maintain adequate ventilation; monitor ABGs, pulse oximetry • Administer IV fluids as ordered (½ to ⅔ maintenance rates) • Monitor for signs of Syndrome of Inappropriate Antidiuretic Hormone (SIADH); restrict fluids if s/s present - low serum Na - low serum osmolarity - oliguria - high urinary Na • Monitor for signs of Diabetes Insipidus - increased urinary output 1-3 L/h - decreased urine osmolarity (urine sp. gr. < 1.005) • Treat Diabetes Insipidus with fluid replacement and administration of DDAVP as ordered
		RATIONALE: *Early detection and prompt management of fluid shifts and electrolyte imbalance prevent further complicating effects of increased ICP.*
3 Altered Tissue Perfusion (cerebral) *r.t. increased ICP, increase in cerebral blood flow producing increased ICP, hemorrhage, brain death*	• Demonstrates no further deterioration in neurologic status	• Assess and monitor neurologic and VS q1-2h (appropriate for age and level of development) - pupils size and response to light - level of consciousness - spontaneous movement/tone

SURGICAL

NURSING DIAGNOSES	OUTCOME CRITERIA	INTERVENTIONS
	• Experiences no complications of increased ICP	• Monitor for signs of increased ICP q1-2h - change in LOC - unequal/sluggish pupil response, change in HR and BP (tachycardia, bradycardia/ hypertension) - irregular breathing pattern (apnea, Cheyne Stokes)
	• Shows no evidence of increased ICP	• Provide measures to control increased ICP - maintain head midline without flexion of neck - HOB up 30° - prevent hypoxemia; maintain PaO_2 80-100 mmHg - monitor electrolytes (prevent fluctuations in Na) - administer diuretic therapy as ordered
	• Sustains no seizure-related obstruction	• Assess and monitor seizure activity - administer anti-epileptic drugs as ordered - position child on side - do not place anything in mouth - maintain airway - monitor and record progression of seizure activity
	• Experiences prompt treatment - seizure activity abates - O_2 sats WNL	• Assess and manage status epilepticus - seizure activity which persists for 20 min or multiple seizures between which the child does not regain consciousness - the intubated and paralyzed child may demonstrate status epilepticus by nystagmus, elevations in ICP monitor readings, fluctuations in VS - administer IV anti-epileptic or sedative drugs as ordered - monitor and anticipate pulmonary compromise (electively intubate if indicated)

RATIONALE: *Early detection and prompt management of complications help to minimize neurologic deterioration.*

NURSING DIAGNOSES	OUTCOME CRITERIA	INTERVENTIONS
4 High Risk for Fluid Volume Deficit *r.t. Diabetes Insipidus, SIADH, fluid restriction, diuretic therapy*	• Demonstrates adequate fluid and electrolyte balance - I&O WNL/restriction - urinary sp. gr. WNL - electrolyte levels appropriate for age - fluid balance appropriate to condition - no rapid changes in weight - flat fontanel (infant) - skin turgor elastic/brisk recoil - capillary refill < 3 sec - intact peripheral pulses	• Monitor I&O - urinary output 1-3 mL/kg/h • Monitor electrolytes; notify physician of abnormal values • Monitor serum osmolarity and urinary sp. gr. • Weigh daily; monitor and report changes (gain or loss) - 50 g/day (infant) - 200 g/day (child) - 500 g/day (adolescent) • Assess and report signs of dehydration - dry mucous membranes - poor skin turgor - sunken fontanel/eyes - monitor for signs of Diabetes Insipidus and SIADH • Assess systemic perfusion - capillary refill, peripheral pulses - skin turgor - fontanel (infant) • Administer IV fluids as ordered • Maintain fluid restrictions as ordered
		RATIONALE: *Providing adequate fluids helps to prevent complications associated with fluid deficit electrolyte imbalance.*
5 Altered Nutrition: Less than body requirements *r.t. inadequate intravenous nutrition, nausea/vomiting, decreased oral intake, gastrointestinal dysfunction*	• Maintains adequate nutritional intake - skin turgor elastic and brisk recoil - moist mucous membranes - stable weight (weight WNL for age)	• Weigh daily • Assess toleration to oral feedings; if no gag reflex, do not PO feed • Provide appropriate diet for age; obtain favorite foods • Do not administer medications with food or favorite fluids • Administer parenteral fluids as ordered
		RATIONALE: *Pediatric patients require high calorie diets.*

SURGICAL

273

NURSING DIAGNOSES	OUTCOME CRITERIA	INTERVENTIONS

6 Ineffective Family Coping
 	
r.t. illness, hospitalization, changes in body image, unknown outcomes
	• Displays minimal anxiety and adequate coping skills
	  - child, parents express understanding of illness, hospital routines, and care
	  - child, parents discuss concerns or questions
	  - continues with ADL within identified limitations
		• Assess parents'/child's knowledge base to disease process and ability to perform ADL
		
		• Provide teaching regarding illness, hospital routines, and use of equipment
		
		• Allow child/parent to verbalize concerns and questions regarding illness and care being provided
		
		• Encourage child/parent participation in care/decision-making when appropriate
		
		• Incorporate home activities with the hospital stay
		
		• Encourage utilization of favorite articles (e.g., toys, blankets) for sense of security
		
		• Consult social work, pastoral care

		RATIONALE: *Knowledge and competence minimize the anxiety of both child and family during hospitalization.*

7 Impaired Skin Integrity
 	
r.t. trauma, surgical wounds
	• Maintains skin integrity
	  - no signs of infection
	  - no CSF leak
		• Assess skin integrity q shift
		
		• Reposition q2h and prn
		
		• Maintain clean dry skin
		
		• Perform passive ROM q shift and prn
		
		• Consult OT/PT
		
		• Notify physician of any bleeding or CSF drainage from wounds, ears, or nose
		
		• Monitor VS; notify physician of temperature > 38°C (100.4°F)

		RATIONALE: *Early detection helps to prevent complications associated with infection and tissue damage.*

NURSING DIAGNOSES	OUTCOME CRITERIA	INTERVENTIONS
8 **High Risk for Injury (external)** *r.t. limited mobility, decreased muscle tone, paralysis, ataxia, seizure activity, neurologic deficit*	• Is free of injury and maintains optimum mobility within constraints of neurologic deficits - maintains ADL - maintains, improves motor capabilities within identified limitations	• Assess (upon admission and ongoing) q4-8h - motor activity - muscle strength - muscle tone • Monitor skin integrity • Maintain extremities in position of function • Reposition q2h and prn • Consult OT/PT to assist with development of plan of care which maximizes child's potential for achievement • Utilize splints and rehabilitative devices as ordered
	• Parents actively participate in care and safety activities	• Instruct child/parents in the importance of maintaining a safe environment (side rails up at all times, supervised play) within the constraints of the child's neurologic deficit • Provide diversional activity for child within neurologic limitations • Encourage active participation in child's ADL; provide stimulation and support to attain difficult tasks
		RATIONALE: *These measures maximize the child's potential for rehabilitation and prevent further deterioration as a result of neurologic deficit.*

SURGICAL

OTHER LESS COMMON NURSING DIAGNOSES: *Altered Urinary Elimination; Pain*

ESSENTIAL DISCHARGE CRITERIA

• Maintains neurologic status within baseline expectations

• Shows surgical wound healing free of infection

• Participates actively in ADL within limitations of neurologic deficit

• Parents acknowledge home care needs and identify community resources to assist/facilitate rehabilitation plans

• Parents verbalize plans for follow-up and list s/s of complications to report to PCP

HIRSCHSPRUNG'S DISEASE, PULL-THROUGH

NURSING DIAGNOSES	OUTCOME CRITERIA	INTERVENTIONS

See "Preoperative" and "Postoperative" care plans

1 High Risk for Impaired Skin Integrity

r.t. frequent acidic stools

- Exhibits no buttock excoriation

- Assess and change diaper q1-2h and prn to remove acidic stool
- Avoid cleansers with alcohol preparation
- Allow buttocks to air-dry following diaper change
- Apply skin ointments prn to protect buttocks from excoriation

RATIONALE: *Cleansing, drying, and ointments protect skin from acid burns, bacterial invasion and proliferation.*

2 High Risk for Injury (bowel obstruction)

r.t. manipulation of bowel during surgery

- Regains peristalsis and bowel function within 72 h of surgery

- Assess bowel status
  - auscultate bowel sound q4h
  - palpate abdomen q4h and record; measure girth prn
  - listen for passage of flatus
- Facilitate return of peristalsis and decrease gaseous distention
  - change position q2h
  - reduce air swallowing
  - increase mobility: out of bed or ambulate q4h
  - maintain patency of nasogastric tube

RATIONALE: *Monitoring bowel function and facilitating its initiation decrease the risk of bowel obstruction.*

3 Diarrhea

r.t. bowel irritation associated with surgery, diet

- Displays minimal abdominal pain, cramping, urgency

- Assess child's behavior for evidence of abdominal pain, cramping q4-8h
- Administer anti-diarrheal medication as ordered

- Passes soft, formed stools; no more than 1-2/day

- Monitor stooling: frequency, color, consistency

NURSING DIAGNOSES	OUTCOME CRITERIA	INTERVENTIONS
	• Parents discuss diet, bowel elimination, toileting	• Teach parents to manage elimination - demonstrate to parents how to observe stools for color, consistency, amount, frequency - explain diet, effects on stools
		RATIONALE: *During the home postoperative period, bowel problems can occur. The parents need to anticipate and manage these side effects.*
4 Knowledge Deficit *r.t. lack of experience with care techniques, follow-up requirements*	• Parents express feelings, ask appropriate questions, perform required care	• Explain expected course of recovery: healing, skin, stooling, skin care
	• Parents select required foods from list	• Review dietary requirements; provide lists to reinforce tracking
	• Parents demonstrate ability to inspect, describe stools	• Review criteria for stool inspection, description
	• Parents list reportable s/s - abdominal pain, fever - bleeding, distention, poor appetite	• Describe, provide list of s/s to report to physician
	• Parents demonstrate confidence in ability to manage care - possess starter supplies - expect one or more home visits from nurse - possess written follow-up appointments	• Support home care - provide dressings and starter supplies for home care - refer for one home visit for support, information - verify possession of follow-up appointments
		RATIONALE: *Knowledgeable, competent parents are likely to effectively manage postoperative care, to detect complications, and to seek timely assistance.*

SURGICAL

> **OTHER LESS COMMON NURSING DIAGNOSES:** *Altered Growth and Development; High Risk for Infection; Urinary Retention*

ESSENTIAL DISCHARGE CRITERIA

- Exhibits no excoriation or healing of buttock skin
- Exhibits initiation/return of bowel function
- Takes 90% of prescribed foods, fluids
- Parents demonstrate understanding of care to maintain skin integrity

- Parents demonstrate competence in child's special care needs
- Parents possess follow-up appointments and list s/s to report to PCP

HYPOSPADIAS REPAIR

NURSING DIAGNOSES	OUTCOME CRITERIA	INTERVENTIONS

See "Preoperative" and "Postoperative" care plans

1 High Risk for Fluid Volume Deficit

r.t. NPO, nausea, vomiting, bleeding

OUTCOME CRITERIA	INTERVENTIONS
• Shows normal VS, BP	• Monitor VS, BP q2-4h x 8h, then q8h
• Shows no bleeding, clots in catheter, or frank bleeding on dressing	• Inspect urine for blood, clots q1-2h x 24h; inspect dressing for bleeding q1-2h x 24h
• Displays moist mucous membranes, good skin turgor	• Assess skin, mucous membranes q2h x 24h
• Exhibits normal respiratory depth, rhythm, rate	• Monitor respirations q2-4h; report if signs of pallor, shallow respirations

RATIONALE: *Frequent monitoring of hydration status prompts timely medical and nursing interventions.*

2 Altered Urinary Elimination

r.t. surgical trauma, catheter clamping

OUTCOME CRITERIA	INTERVENTIONS
• Shows urinary output WNL by 24h post-op	• Maintain strict I&O
• Voids spontaneously by 8h post catheter removal; urine clearing, clear	• Monitor output qh x 8 then q2h • Check patency, inspect color of drainage q4-8h • Irrigate per orders q4-8h • Assess abdomen for bladder distension, pain

RATIONALE: *Frequent monitoring of urinary drainage prompts early detection and timely management of catheter patency.*

3 Pain

r.t. surgical procedure, catheter

OUTCOME CRITERIA	INTERVENTIONS
• Exhibits signs of decreasing pain - less crying - decreased restlessness - fewer complaints of pain	• Administer analgesics as ordered prn • Assess for pain and/or pain relief q2-3h • Assess for incisional pain vs. bladder spasms

SURGICAL

NURSING DIAGNOSES	OUTCOME CRITERIA	INTERVENTIONS
	• Displays no guarding of surgical area	• Check catheter and/or stent position q diaper change
		• Avoid pressure to surgical site when picking child up (don't straddle child on hip)
		RATIONALE: *Medicating for pain increases comfort and decreases anxiety. Positioning of stent and child to decrease movement of stent will decrease pain.*

4 High Risk for Infection
 	
r.t. placement of indwelling catheter and/or stent in urinary tract
	• Exhibits no s/s of infection
	  - VS WNL
	  - clear, odorless urine
	  - no flank pain
	  - no foul odor, purulent drainage, swelling
		• Administer prophylactic antibiotics as ordered

		• Monitor VS q4h
		• Observe urine for characteristics of infections: cloudiness, sedimentation, and odor
		• Observe for flank pain
		• Monitor surgical dressing for foul odor, purulent drainage, or unusual swelling
		• Use aseptic technique in manipulating and emptying catheter and stent
		• Cleanse stent as ordered using aseptic technique
		• Keep any urine collection bag below bladder level
		• Avoid kinks and loops in drainage tubing
		• Encourage patient to drink fluids in excess of minimal requirement
		RATIONALE: *Minimize the introduction of bacteria into open sites and avoid urinary stasis, which would create a medium for bacterial multiplication.*

NURSING DIAGNOSES	OUTCOME CRITERIA	INTERVENTIONS

5 High Risk for Injury (internal, external)
 	
r.t. post-op bleeding
	• Shows no s/s of bleeding or injury
	  - VS WNL
	  - maintains urinary output WNL
	  - does not tug, pull at catheter/stent
	  - exhibits no guarding
		• Observe for bleeding with every diaper change q3-4h
		
		• Monitor VS q4h
		
		• Maintain double diaper technique with stent and penis pointing upward toward the abdomen with ventral side up; use gentle care in placing or removing stent through diaper opening
		
		• Restrain hands and legs as necessary
		
		• Notify surgeon if bleeding occurs or stent is displaced

		RATIONALE: *Trauma-induced bleeding can be a complication of hypospadias repair.*
6 Knowledge Deficit *r.t. inexperience with care techniques; concern about complications, cosmetic, functional results*	• Parents discuss expected course of recovery, ask appropriate questions	• Teach, discuss surgical anatomy, expected course of recovery, treatment rationale
	• Parents demonstrate required catheter, incisional care	• Instruct parents to care for catheter and/or stent in penis, including any cleansing around the stent; how to give baths, empty the drainage bag, secure the catheter, and double-diaper the infant • Explain activity limitations
	• Parents demonstrate ability to assess urine: amount, color, consistency • Parents list reportable s/s: fever, cloudy urine, drainage, foul smell	• Instruct parents or caregiver on s/s of urinary tract or incisional infection
	• Parents discuss medications: antibiotics, analgesics; discuss effects, side effects	• Explain any antibiotics or analgesics: effects, side effects, dosages, times to administer
	• Parents discuss concerns about cosmetic and functional outcome of surgery; understand need to ask surgeon about unresolved questions	• Listen to parents' perceptions; refer to surgeon to resolve concerns about ultimate cosmetic, functional results

SURGICAL

NURSING DIAGNOSES	OUTCOME CRITERIA	INTERVENTIONS
	• Parents possess follow-up appointments	• Verify parents' knowledge of follow-up appointments and physician's phone number for questions

RATIONALE: *Parents' knowledge, care skills, and the ability to express and resolve concerns foster their becoming competent caregivers at home.*

OTHER LESS COMMON NURSING DIAGNOSES: *Sleep Pattern Disturbance; Anxiety*

ESSENTIAL DISCHARGE CRITERIA

- Exhibits clean incision
- Urine is free of bleeding, clots, sediment
- Takes 90% of required nutrition

- Parents demonstrate required catheter, incisional care and ability to inspect, describe urine output
- Parents verbalize knowledge of expected follow-up schedule with physician

MASTOIDECTOMY

See "Preoperative" and "Postoperative" care plans

1 High Risk for Fluid Volume Deficit

r.t. hypovolemia associated with perioperative bleeding

- Remains free of bright red drainage on dressing

- Detect, minimize bleeding
  - inspect dressing at least qh
  - reinforce if bleeding, drainage
  - report any bleeding, drainage through dressing
  - be aware that only the physician will change dressing
  - elevate HOB
  - position child on unoperated side

RATIONALE: *Frequent inspections and prompt, early detection of bleeding in this highly vascular area of the head are essential.*

---

2 High Risk for Injury (internal)

r.t. facial nerve damage associated with surgical trauma

- Wrinkles forehead, puckers lips, bares grimace by post-op Day 2

- Ask child to pucker, grimace, close eyes q2-4h x 24h

- Has no difficulty with swallowing by post-op Day 2

- Observe swallowing for any difficulty

- Shows no facial edema by post-op Day 2

- Inspect face for edema q2-4h; report any facial changes

- Administer ordered corticosteroids; assess effects, side effects

RATIONALE: *Frequent inspection provides comparison data.*

---

3 Pain

r.t. surgical trauma

- Verbalizes, displays reasonable comfort; has no prolonged moaning, crying, restlessness

- Perform a comprehensive assessment of pain utilizing age-appropriate pediatric assessment tools; document q2-4h

SURGICAL

NURSING DIAGNOSES	OUTCOME CRITERIA	INTERVENTIONS

	• Exhibits relaxed body posture, facial expression
	
	• Exhibits no guarding, pulling at dressing
	
	• Smiles, interacts
		• Control pain; provide comfort measures
		  - administer ordered analgesics; assess effects, side effects
		  - provide quiet play activities, music, television, soft toys
		  - include parents in soothing, diversional activities

		RATIONALE: *Comfort aids healing and minimizes child's pulling at dressing.*
4 Knowledge Deficit *r.t. parents' inexperience with home care, potential complications*	• Parents discuss surgical anatomy, ask appropriate questions, demonstrate dressing care	• Review, discuss surgical anatomy, rationale for treatment, required care techniques
	• Parents verbalize knowledge of adverse s/s: fever, agitation, vomiting, disorientation, headache	• Discuss, provide list of potential s/s
	• Parents express commitment to consistent follow-up to treat, prevent otitis media; possess follow-up appointments	• Provide phone numbers for emergency, routine follow-up care • Review need for faithful follow-up, for both near- and long-term • Verify knowledge of appointments
		RATIONALE: *Knowledgeable, competent parents are highly likely to foster a successful recovery at home.*

OTHER LESS COMMON NURSING DIAGNOSES: *Anxiety; High Risk for Infection; Altered Nutrition: Less than body requirements*

ESSENTIAL DISCHARGE CRITERIA

• Surgical site healing; no signs of infection

• Takes 90% of required nutrition

• Parents demonstrate correct dressing care

• Parents verbalize plan for follow-up treatment, prevention of otitis media

NEUROBLASTOMA, SURGICAL REPAIR

NURSING DIAGNOSES	OUTCOME CRITERIA	INTERVENTIONS

See "Preoperative" and "Postoperative" care plans

1 High Risk for Infection

r.t. suppressed immune system secondary to neoplasm

- Remains free of s/s of infection
  - VS WNL
  - surgical wound without redness, swelling, or drainage
  - WBC WNL

- Provide information and education preoperatively on coughing, turning, and deep breathing
- Implement universal precautions with all body fluids
- Assess for s/s of infection at surgical site
  - inflammation
  - warmth
  - bleeding
  - purulent drainage
- Utilize aseptic technique during dressing changes; change dressing as ordered to maintain a dry, intact dressing
- Document wound condition q2-4h and at dressing changes
- Administer all prophylactic antibiotics within scheduled administration time
- Provide information and education on appropriate aseptic practices
- Protect from sources of infection
  - provide private room
  - provide education on hand-washing
  - limit visitation if appropriate
  - screen visitors for known infections or recent exposure to infections
  - limit invasive procedures

- Maintains temperature < 38°C (100.4°F)

- Monitor temperature q4h; notify physician if elevated
- Assess nutritional status; provide adequate protein and calorie intake

- Shows lab work WNL

- Evaluate lab studies, CBC, culture and sensitivities
- Notify physician and/or infectious disease coordinator of abnormal lab studies

SURGICAL

285

NURSING DIAGNOSES	OUTCOME CRITERIA	INTERVENTIONS
	• Parents verbalize compliance with immunization schedule for age	• Assess for adequate immunizations against childhood diseases, bacterial infections, and other viral infections
		RATIONALE: *Potentially life-threatening infections can occur in children who are immuno-compromised due to neuroblastoma or chemotherapy treatment.*
2 Pain *r.t. surgical incision*	• Achieves adequate pain control - verbal statement of comfort - absence of guarding behavior - appropriate social response to parents and friends - adequate periods of sleep and rest	• Provide information, education concerning sources of pain • Acknowledge child's pain; assure him/her that you are assessing their pain so you can help reduce it • Provide periods for rest during the day and periods of uninterrupted sleep at night • Utilize alternative pain reduction methods such as distraction • Medicate prior to activities • Consult with physician for increased pain medication at bedtime, if needed - administer ordered analgesic; assess VS (especially RR) prior to administering analgesia - instruct child to request prn pain medication before pain is too severe - collaborate with physician in planning 24-h analgesia rather than prn - assess the response to the pain relief medication
		RATIONALE: *Reduction of pain in the child who has undergone abdominal surgery permits increased participation in activities and reduction in anxiety.*

NURSING DIAGNOSES	OUTCOME CRITERIA	INTERVENTIONS

3 Activity Intolerance
 	
r.t. presence of neuroblastoma and/or recent abdominal surgery
	• Progresses activity to accomplish ADL without excessive fatigue
	  - naps as needed
		• Reduce or eliminate contributing factors to fatigue
		  - pain
		  - inadequate rest or sleep periods
		  - stress/anxiety
		  - medication side effects
		• Provide rest periods after periods of increased activity
		• Plan daily schedule with child and parents
		• Consult Child Life specialist

	• Reports/demonstrates activity tolerance
	  - VS WNL
	  - participates willingly in care activities
		• Monitor child's response to increased activity
		  - obtain resting VS for comparison
		  - obtain post-activity VS
		  - stop activity if child experiences dizziness, bradycardia, hypotension, respiratory distress
		• Increase activity gradually
		  - begin with ROM exercises
		  - obtain physical/occupational therapy consult
		  - slowly increase child's performance of ADL
		  - increase time out of bed each day

	• Parents initiate ideas for fostering activity tolerance; participate in care activities	• Allow child/parents to verbalize their feelings regarding decreased activity tolerance • Provide information regarding methods of increasing activity tolerance and/or the use of assistive devices

RATIONALE: *Promote participation in activities that assist in achieving a level of activity that is desired by both the patient and the health care team.*

SURGICAL

NURSING DIAGNOSES	OUTCOME CRITERIA	INTERVENTIONS
4 Anxiety *r.t. recent diagnosis of neuroblastoma, impending surgery and/or antineoplastic therapy*	• Parent/child display appropriate coping mechanisms - report decreased anxiety	• Assess anxiety levels of child/parents • Provide reassurance, comfort - stay with family - do not request decisions if child/parents are acutely anxious - support present coping mechanisms without confronting defenses or rationalizations - reorient to reality as required - respect personal space - speak slowly and calmly • Decrease sensory stimulation - provide quiet, nonstimulating environment - use short, simple sentences - give clear, concise directions - provide written material to reinforce discussion • Establish trusting relationship
	• Parents/family maintain sustained schedule of child visitation	• Minimize child's separation from parents • Encourage expression of fears and feelings • Encourage parental involvement in care • Reduce and help modify problematic coping mechanisms

RATIONALE: *Children's anxieties are heightened by separation from parents, routine changes, strange environments, painful procedures, and parental anxiety.*

> **OTHER LESS COMMON NURSING DIAGNOSES:** Ineffective Breathing Pattern;
> Ineffective Family Coping: Compromised

ESSENTIAL DISCHARGE CRITERIA

- Incision healing and is free of s/s of infection
- Achieves progressive activity levels
- Shows evidence of adaptive coping and reduced anxiety
- Patient/parent verbalize plans for home care, demonstrate required treatments
- Parents verbalize plans for follow-up and list s/s of complications to report to PCP

SURGICAL

ORTHOPEDIC REPAIR, LIMB FRACTURE

NURSING DIAGNOSES	OUTCOME CRITERIA	INTERVENTIONS

See "Preoperative" and "Postoperative" care plans

1 Impaired Physical Mobility

r.t. fracture, surgical procedure, fixation device

• Maintains optimal age-appropriate physical mobility (within limits of fracture and treatment)	• Adapt age-appropriate play activities to imposed restrictions
• Exhibits normal ROM of unaffected joints, limbs	• Provide active and passive ROM qid
• Achieves relative freedom of movement	• Use equipment to mobilize child (bed, gurney, buggy, wagon, stroller, wheelchair)

RATIONALE: *Play promotes movement and normalcy. Regular activity maintains muscle strength and joint motion. Mobility options simulate usual activity.*

2 Pain

r.t. fracture, muscle spasm, soft tissue injury/repair

• Verbalizes, displays freedom from pain - reports comfort - displays relaxed body posture, facial expression - no guarding - no extended crying	• Assess pain accurately at each age level • Provide regularly scheduled analgesia with prn supplement • Medicate prior to pain-promoting activities and therapies • Keep affected part immobile • Elevate affected part above level of heart • Apply cold first 24-48h for 20 min q1-2h • Support, position, reposition unaffected parts q2h

RATIONALE: *Immobilization prevents muscle spasm and further tissue damage. Cold decreases vasocongestion/edema. Supported position change promotes general comfort, prevents pressure areas.*

NURSING DIAGNOSES	OUTCOME CRITERIA	INTERVENTIONS
3 High Risk for Injury *r.t. trauma, surgery, neurovascular compromise, altered peripheral tissue perfusion*	• Maintains tissue perfusion in both affected and unaffected extremities - color, motion, and sensitivity WNL - pulses present and strong - capillary refill < 3 sec	• Elevate affected part; apply cold • Monitor constricting properties of fixation device • Monitor color, motion, and sensitivity; pulses, capillary refill qh, then q2-4h • Report abnormal findings promptly
		RATIONALE: *Early detection/management of altered tissue perfusion distal to fracture prevents injury.*
4 High Risk for Infection *r.t. surgery and/or fixation device*	• Remains free of local infections - no redness - no edema - no warmth - no drainage • Is free of signs of systemic infection - no fever of > 38.4°C (100.4°F) after first post-op day - exhibits WBC WNL - no delayed healing	• Assess for local and systemic signs of infection q2-4h first 48h post surgery, then q8h
	• Has no odors from drainage around or through fixation device	• Perform pin-site care per institutional protocol • Keep all dressings dry and intact • Administer topical, oral, and parenteral antibiotics properly
		RATIONALE: *Frequent monitoring fosters early detection/management of infection. The measures described prevent microorganisms from multiplying/reaching wound.*

SURGICAL

NURSING DIAGNOSES	OUTCOME CRITERIA	INTERVENTIONS

5 Knowledge Deficit
 	
r.t. inexperience with orthopedic care techniques
	• Parents/child verbalize/demonstrate knowledge regarding
	  - mobility limitations and safety
	  - adaptations to facilitate ADLs (including school participation)
	  - maintenance of fixation device
	  - signs of possible complications
	  - plans for follow-up care
		• Encourage questions from parents, child, and siblings
		
		• Determine understanding of fracture and treatment; clarify misconceptions
		
		• Assess ability to care for child and provide access to support services (including school)
		
		• Evaluate return demonstration of home care skills
		
		• Instruct parents/child in
		  - positions to increase circulation, decrease edema
		  - exercises to maintain ROM and muscle tone
		  - pain control
		  - nutrition that fosters healing and elimination
		  - acquisition and use of mobility devices (wheelchair, car, restraint, crutches)
		  - signs of neurovascular compromise
		  - plan for follow-up care
		
		• Instruct parents/child in management of fixation device
		  - pin and wound care
		  - signs of infections
		  - protection and care of device
		
		• Instruct parents/child in management of cast

RATIONALE: *Teaching that involves the learner and is directed toward a felt need results in effective learning and competency.*

> ***OTHER LESS COMMON NURSING DIAGNOSES:*** *High Risk for Fluid Volume Deficit; Constipation; Altered Nutrition: Less than body requirements; Ineffective Breathing Pattern; High Risk for Impaired Skin Integrity*

ESSENTIAL DISCHARGE CRITERIA

- Possesses and demonstrates means of mobility
- Requires minimal medication for pain control
- Displays normal peripheral tissue perfusion in affected/unaffected limb(s)

- Is free of signs of infection
- Patient/parents show mastery of required home care
- Parents verbalize plans for follow-up and list s/s of complications to report to PCP

SURGICAL

PYLORIC STENOSIS REPAIR

NURSING DIAGNOSES	OUTCOME CRITERIA	INTERVENTIONS

See "Preoperative" and "Postoperative" care plans

1 High Risk for Fluid Volume Deficit

r.t. vomiting

- Maintains normal, balanced I&O
  - Maintain strict I&O
    - assess fluid balance

- Has normal urinary sp. gr., serum electrolytes
  - Test urinary sp. gr. q4-8h
    - monitor serum electrolytes

- Exhibits good skin turgor, moist mucous membranes, normal fontanel tension
  - Assess skin, mucous membranes, fontanels q4-8h

- Maintains body weight at baseline
  - Weigh daily, same scale

- Has no evidence of abdominal distention; emesis minimal, absent
  - Observe, record vomitus: frequency, amount, color, characteristics; presence, absence of projectile emesis
  - Inspect, palpate abdomen for distention q2-4h
  - Insert ordered nasogastric tube for vomiting, distention

RATIONALE: *Monitoring/managing gastric distention reduces vomiting. Attention to I&O provides opportunity for early identification and treatment of deficit.*

2 Altered Nutrition: Less than body requirements

r.t. vomiting, gradual reintroduction of feedings

- Maintains body weight that is at least 90% of ideal
- Shows consistent weight gain
  - Weigh daily
    - plot weight for age

- Exhibits no abdominal distention
  - Monitor for vomiting, distention; if present, hold feedings, report

- Takes at least 90% of ordered feeds; takes oral feedings without vomiting
  - Maintain required nutritional intake:
    - slowly graduate oral feedings from clear liquid, liquid, soft per orders
    - feed slowly; burp often
    - use infant seat for positioning
    - administer ordered parenteral feedings; assess effects

NURSING DIAGNOSES	OUTCOME CRITERIA	INTERVENTIONS
	• Parents perform feedings • Parents discuss rationale for techniques	• Include parents in feeding techniques; demonstrate, explain reasons for position, slow feedings, burping
		RATIONALE: *Monitoring/maintaining required nutritional intake fosters adequate weight gain and nutrition*
3 Pain *r.t. surgical trauma*	• Verbalizes, displays comfort - no prolonged crying, restlessness - sleeps, naps qs	• Assess for s/s of pain q2-4h • Administer pain medication as indicated
	• Displays behaviors consistent with comfort - no resistance to holding, cuddling, rocking - no undue crying, moaning, restlessness, rigidity, listlessness	• Rock, cuddle, offer pacifier frequently • Include parents in soothing behaviors • Cleanse mouth frequently for comfort • Provide diversions appropriate for age
		RATIONALE: *Controlling pain results in faster recovery. Healing is accelerated, and there is better tolerance for feeding.*
4 Knowledge Deficit *r.t. inexperience, fear of recurrence*	• Parents discuss surgical anatomy, rationale for treatment; ask appropriate questions	• Discuss surgical anatomy, rationale for surgery, prognosis - provide diagram of anatomy
	• Parents demonstrate correct feeding techniques	• Demonstrate feeding techniques; obtain successful return demonstration
	• Parents participate in care	• Include parents in plan of care
	• Parents demonstrate successful soothing, cuddling, rocking techniques	• Allow parents to soothe, rock child
	• Parents list reportable s/s: weight loss, vomiting, fever, abdominal distention, rigidity, restlessness, lethargy	• Review, provide list of reportable s/s

SURGICAL

NURSING DIAGNOSES	OUTCOME CRITERIA	INTERVENTIONS
	• Parents possess written follow-up appointments	• Refer to community resource people for help with difficulties; verify possession of written follow-up appointments
		RATIONALE: *Educating parents increases their skills, self-confidence, and knowledge, resulting in a successful postoperative recovery at home.*

OTHER LESS COMMON NURSING DIAGNOSES: *Altered Family Processes; Fear*

ESSENTIAL DISCHARGE CRITERIA

- Takes and retains at least 90% of oral feedings
- Maintains, shows weight gain

- Parents demonstrate successful feeding, soothing, incision care techniques
- Parents verbalize plans for follow-up and list s/s to report to PCP

NURSING DIAGNOSES	OUTCOME CRITERIA	INTERVENTIONS

See "Preoperative" and "Postoperative" care plans

1 Anxiety

r.t. preoperative fear of surgical risks, prognoses, unfamiliar postoperative care

• Parents discuss accurate knowledge of prognosis	• Listen for misperceptions, inappropriate reactions; clarify, provide information
• Parents/child make realistic statements about expected course of recovery, prognosis	• Explain rationale for surgery, expected course of recovery
• Parents identify support person(s)	• Verify that parents have support person(s)
	RATIONALE: *Stress and anxiety are reduced when information and support are provided.*

2 High Risk for Fluid Volume Deficit

r.t. perioperative bleeding, parenteral fluids, altered kidney function

• Shows normal VS; acceptable BP (not over 95% of normal for age)	• Monitor VS, BP q1-2h post-op Days 1-3, then q2-4h when stable; monitor CVP if line in
• Has urine output of 3-5 mL/kg/h; shows no frank bleeding by post-op Days 3-4	• Measure, inspect urine per VS schedule
• Shows serum electrolytes, BUN normalizing, stable	• Monitor electrolytes • Administer IV fluids as ordered
• Shows stable body weight	• Weigh daily
	RATIONALE: *Careful monitoring of hydration is required for early detection and prompt management of either fluid deficit or excess.*

3 High Risk for Infection

r.t. surgical invasion

• Is afebrile	• Monitor body temperature q1-2h post-op Days 1-3 then q2-4h; report if over 38.5°C (101°F)
• Displays no swelling, redness, warmth around wound; no cloudy, purulent wound drainage	• Inspect wound, change dressing q8h and per unit protocols

SURGICAL

297

NURSING DIAGNOSES	OUTCOME CRITERIA	INTERVENTIONS
	• Is free of urinary cloudiness or foul odor	• Maintain strict I&O; measure, inspect all drainage q8h
		RATIONALE: *Because of cortisone therapy for renal disease the child's immune system is suppressed. Frequent monitoring for infection is necessary for prompt detection and management.*
4 Altered Tissue Perfusion (renal) *r.t. kidney disease, fluid volume excess*	• Maintains body temperature < 38.0°C (100.4°F); BP normal for age and condition	• Monitor body temperature, BP q1-2h post-op Days 1-3 then q2-4h
	• Shows urinary output > 3-5 mL/kg/h	• Monitor urinary output q1-2h post-op Days 1-3 then q2-4h
	• Achieves weight gain of < 1 kg/d	• Weigh daily
	• Displays no edema	• Inspect for peripheral, periorbital edema
		RATIONALE: *Preoperative kidney disease compounded by surgery puts added stress on renal function.*
5 Pain *r.t. flank incision, invasive procedures*	• Verbalizes, displays reasonable comfort - relaxed body posture, facial expression - smiles, plays, interacts - sleeps, naps qs - no moaning, guarding - ambulates on schedule without undue resistance	• Assess level of pain q2-4h; administer ordered analgesics; assess relief, side effects • Provide comfort measures - provide distraction, diversion, back rubs, holding, massage, favorite soft toys - provide uninterrupted nap, sleep periods - explain all invasive procedures to parents, child before initiating
		RATIONALE: *Consistent, anticipatory pain management measures provide for sustained comfort.*

NURSING DIAGNOSES	OUTCOME CRITERIA	INTERVENTIONS
6 Knowledge Deficit *r.t. lack of information regarding complications, activity levels*	• Parents/child discuss expected course of recovery, ask appropriate questions	• Discuss surgical anatomy, rationale for treatment, expected course of recovery
	• Parents demonstrate required wound care	• Demonstrate required wound care; have parents provide return demonstration
	• Parents verbalize knowledge of complications: edema; fever; tenderness, swelling over surgical area; cloudy urine	• Review reportable s/s; explain significance
	• Parents verbalize knowledge of medications: effects, side effects	• Review medications: effects, side effects, dosages
	• Parents/child express confidence in ability to manage care	• Listen to parents' fears, concerns
	• Parents express commitment to consistent medical follow-ups	• Review need for consistent medical follow-up; verify knowledge of follow-up appointments

RATIONALE: *Knowledgeable, committed parents are likely to manage a safe, uneventful recovery at home.*

SURGICAL

OTHER LESS COMMON NURSING DIAGNOSES: *Activity Intolerance; Altered Family Processes*

ESSENTIAL DISCHARGE CRITERIA

- Is afebrile
- Shows no extreme variations in lab values
- Shows minimal or no edema

- Has stabilized body weight
- Parents verbalize, demonstrate home care requirements and list potential complications to report to PCP

TRACHEOSTOMY

NURSING DIAGNOSES	OUTCOME CRITERIA	INTERVENTIONS

See "Preoperative" and "Postoperative" care plans

1 Ineffective Airway Clearance

r.t. presence of secretions, potential for tube dislodgement

- Maintains effective breathing patterns

- Encourage child to cough to clear secretions; suction when child cannot clear own secretions
  - suction only length of tracheostomy tube
  - may suction past distal cannula per unit standards

- Administer humidity to environment and PO fluids

- Apply humidivent to tracheostomy while child is ambulatory

- Clean inner cannula per hospital protocol tid with half-strength H_2O_2 and trach brush; rinse thoroughly and dry (disposable inner cannulas are changed qd; they are not to be reused)

- Maintains proper placement of tracheostomy tube

- Change tube ties daily and secure per hospital protocol
  - secure ties with triple square knot (use no bows); check ties q2-4h to ensure fit
  - obturator for tube should be taped over head of bed
  - keep a spare tube of same size at the bedside with obturator and ties in place
  - keep an emergency tube that is one size smaller than child's prepared as above at the bed side
  - keep scissors, curved hemostat, and extra ties at the bed side

RATIONALE: *Frequent coughing, suctioning oral fluids, and humidified air reduce viscosity of tracheal fluids, making it easier to clear secretions. Meticulous cleaning of cannulas keeps airway patent. Protection of tube placement and emergency preparation for dislodgement protect the child from airway closure secondary to tube displacement.*

NURSING DIAGNOSES	OUTCOME CRITERIA	INTERVENTIONS
2 High Risk for Injury (hypoxia) *r.t. suctioning, mucous plugs*	• Remains free from hypoxia - exhibits no s/s of cyanosis - maintains O_2 sats WNL	• Assess need for increased O_2 or hyperventilation for non-ventilator-dependent children; if needed, administer 4-5 manual breaths prior to suctioning • Provide ventilator-dependent children with 5 manual or mechanical breaths and/or increased O_2 with suctioning, and give an additional 5 breaths and time for recovery between suction passes • Use catheter with diameter no more than one-half the diameter of the trach tube • Apply suction for no more than 5 seconds
		RATIONALE: *Maintaining a clear, patent airway minimizes the potential for hypoxia.*
3 High Risk for Impaired Skin Integrity *r.t. moisture from secretions and humidity, mechanical irritation, infections around tracheostomy*	• Achieves, maintains intact external stomal skin without evidence of breakdown or infection	• Cleanse stomal area tid with half-strength H_2O_2 per hospital protocol • Cleanse excoriated stomal skin with ¼-strength acetic acid • Dry area thoroughly after cleaning • Change fenestrated drain sponges prn when wet or soiled (fenestrated drain sponges may be used only with extreme caution, as they obstruct view of the trach site and may hinder early detection of decannulation)
		RATIONALE: *Cleansing with H_2O_2 debrides dead tissue from area. Acetic acid creates a low pH in area, thus decreasing bacterial growth.*

SURGICAL

NURSING DIAGNOSES	OUTCOME CRITERIA	INTERVENTIONS

4 Altered Oral Mucous Membrane
 	
r.t. suctioning, friction from tracheostomy tube
	• Maintains optimal tracheal mucosal integrity; absence of bleeding and granulation tissue	• Suction child only when needed
		  - use calibrated suction catheter
		  - suction only length of tube
		  - use catheters with open tips and a minimum of one side vent
		  - apply suction only when withdrawing the catheter
		
		• Check vacuum prior to each suction episode; vacuum should be set at 80-120 mm or per unit standards
		
		• Report frank, bright red bleeding

		RATIONALE: *Gentle suctioning, a safe amount of vacuum, and inspection for bleeding prevent tissue damage and granulation.*
5 Impaired Verbal Communication *r.t. inability to vocalize needs*	• Communicates needs to caregivers and significant others	• Provide consultation to speech/language pathologist • Assist with implementation of augmented communication system • Assist family/child to evaluate effectiveness of augmented communication system
		RATIONALE: *Creating nonverbal ways to communicate reduces child's fear and frustrations.*

6 Knowledge Deficit
 	
r.t. inexperience with care of child with tracheostomy
	• Parents/child demonstrate the following skills
	  - suctioning
	  - stomal skin care
	  - inner cannula care
	  - tie change
	  - tube change
	  - CPR and emergency measures
		• Teach a minimum of two adults how to manage tracheostomy care
		
		• Teach skills in a progressive order, going from easiest (skin care) to most difficult (tube change)
		
		• Provide verbal support and reinforcement
		
		• Encourage parent/child to assume responsibility for providing hands-on care as they learn each skill
		
		• Provide parents/child with written instructions for each skill

NURSING DIAGNOSES	OUTCOME CRITERIA	INTERVENTIONS
		• Initiate community health nurse referral
		• Assist family in arranging follow-up care

RATIONALE: *Directed learning, positive support, and discussion of care increase competency and confidence.*

OTHER LESS COMMON NURSING DIAGNOSES: *Altered Nutrition: Less than body requirements; Pain (acute, chronic); Caregiver Role Strain*

ESSENTIAL DISCHARGE CRITERIA

• Displays good oxygenation, good skin color, pink mucous membranes with no s/s of infection

• Takes 90% of required nutrition

• Two adults demonstrate ability to provide tracheostomy care and verbalize plan for emergency situations

• Parents have follow-up care with pediatrician and otolaryngologist arranged

SURGICAL

303

VENTRICULAR SHUNT REVISION

NURSING DIAGNOSES	OUTCOME CRITERIA	INTERVENTIONS

See "Preoperative" and "Postoperative" care plans

1 High Risk for Infection

r.t. surgical invasion, immunosuppression

- Remains free of infection
  - wound healing without redness or purulent drainage
  - normothermia

- Monitor VS and perform neuro checks q2h; report any changes to the physician
- Observe surgical incision for redness, swelling, or purulent drainage
- Utilize aseptic technique when changing dressing
- Administer antibiotics as ordered; assess effects, side effects

RATIONALE: *Any invasion of tissue increases risk of microbial invasion. Frequent monitoring for s/s of infection fosters prompt intervention.*

2 High Risk for Impaired Skin Integrity

r.t. surgical procedure, increased ICP, decreased movement

- Displays clear, intact skin

- Massage bony prominences q2-4h; teach parents to provide this treatment
- Place sheep skin padding beneath the patient's head
- Reposition the patient's head and extremities q2h, except when contraindicated
- Do not position the patient on operative side until a physician's order is obtained

RATIONALE: *Pressure areas with associated limited arterial/venous circulation produce friability and breakdown of skin. Repositioning, careful massage minimize pressure areas, improve circulation.*

NURSING DIAGNOSES	OUTCOME CRITERIA	INTERVENTIONS

3 High Risk for Injury
 	
r.t. potential shunt obstructions (kinking/plugging, thrombosis, displacement)
	• Displays shunt patency
	  - draining of ventricles through shunt
	  - prompt refilling of ventricular chamber
	  - ICP ranges between 5-15 mmHg
		• Test the valve for patency when ordered; repeat when indicated or as ordered
		• Notify physician if pump is difficult to depress
		• Maintain HOB slightly elevated

	• Exhibits none of following s/s of increased ICP
	  - changes in LOC
	  - changes in VS (widening pulse pressure, decreased pulse rate)
	  - restlessness, irritability
	  - headache
	  - vomiting
	  - bulging fontanels
	  - ataxia
	  - sensory loss
		• Perform a thorough neurologic exam per unit standards; carefully observe for signs of increased ICP; repeat q1-2h

	• Parents/child express understanding of shunt and monitoring procedures
	  - ask questions
	  - discuss physiology of shunt
	  - report observations, seek clarification
		• Explain all procedures in simple terms
		• Reinforce/repeat all instructions each time parent participates in care
		• Encourage frequent visitation

		RATIONALE: *Mechanical difficulties such as kinking, plugging, thrombosis, displacement or exudate in the tubing, can obstruct the shunt causing an increase in ICP.*
4 Knowledge Deficit; Anxiety *r.t. hospitalization, illness, uncertain prognosis*	• Parents/child express concerns about illness, hospitalization	• Assign primary nurse to provide continuity in care • Instruct parents/child about illness, hospital routines, and equipment • Provide factual information about child's condition • Include child in some decision-making if developmentally appropriate
	• Parents demonstrate safe, effective care of child	• Encourage parental participation in care

SURGICAL

NURSING DIAGNOSES	OUTCOME CRITERIA	INTERVENTIONS
	• Provide parents/child with pertinent literature regarding ventricular shunts	• Provide sessions with parents to instruct them on s/s of infection, shunt malfunction, and increased ICP
	• Parents identify specific community resources that can be of help	• Provide referrals to community resources
		• Ensure parents understand all instruction prior to discharge

RATIONALE: *Parents' knowledge and competence reduce anxiety and increase likelihood of a safe, uneventful recovery at home.*

OTHER LESS COMMON NURSING DIAGNOSES:
Altered Family Processes; Knowledge Deficit; Fluid Volume Deficit

---

ESSENTIAL DISCHARGE CRITERIA

• Manifests normal neurologic status

• Shows no evidence of systemic or local infection

• Parents demonstrate safe, effective care techniques

• Parents identify plan for follow-up, list s/s of complications to report to PCP

APPENDIXES

CONTENTS

APPENDIXES

APPENDIX A: ABBREVIATIONS

Abbreviations used in this book

ABG(s)	arterial blood gases	**h**	hour	**PCO₂**	partial arterial pressure, carbon dioxide
ADL(s)	activities of daily living	**Hb**	hemoglobin	**PCP**	primary care provider
AIDS	acquired immunodeficiency syndrome	**Hct**	hematocrit	**PERL**	pupils equal and reactive to light
ANC	absolute neutrophil count	**Hg**	mercury		
AP	apical pulse	**HIV**	human immunodificiency virus	**pH**	measure of acidity
ASAP	as soon as possible	**H₂O₂**	hydrogen peroxide	**PO**	orally, by mouth
		HOB	head of bed	**PO₂**	partial arterial pressure, oxygen
bid	twice daily	**hpf**	high power field	**PRBC**	packed red blood cells
BP	blood pressure	**HR**	heart rate	**prn**	as needed
bpm	beats per minute			**PT**	prothrombin time
BUN	blood urea nitrogen	**ICP**	intracranial pressure	**PT**	physical therapy
		ID	identification	**PTT**	partial prothrombin time
C	centigrade	**IM**	intramuscular	**PVC**	premature ventricular contraction
Ca	calcium	**I&O**	intake and output		
CBC	complete blood count	**ISADH**	inappropriate secretion of antidiuretic hormone	**q**	every
cc	cubic centimeter	**IV**	intravenous	**qd**	every day
CDC	communicable disease controls	**IVIG**	intravenous gamma globulin	**qh**	every hour
CF	cystic fibrosis			**qid**	four times daily
CHF	congestive heart failure	**JRA**	juvenile rheumatoid arthritis	**qs**	quantity sufficient
CHO	carbohydrate				
cm	centimeter	**K**	potassium	**RBC**	red blood cells
CMV	cytomegalovirus	**kg**	kilogram	**ROM**	range of motion
CNS	central nervous system			**RR**	respiratory rate
CO₂	carbon dioxide	**L**	liter	**r.t.**	related to
CP	cerebral palsy	**lab**	laboratory	**Rx**	prescription
CPP	cerebral perfusion pressure	**lb**	pound		
CPPD	clapping, percussion, postural drainage	**LOC**	level of consciousness	**SaO₂**	oxygen saturation
CPR	cardiopulmonary resuscitation			**sec**	second(s)
CPT	chest physiotherapy	**mEq**	millequivalents	**SGA**	small for gestational age
CRT	capillary refill time	**min**	minutes	**SIADH**	syndrome of inappropriate antidiuretic hormone
CSF	cerebrospinal fluid	**mg**	microgrem		
CVP	central venous pressure	**mL**	milliliters	**SIDS**	sudden infant death syndrome
		mm	millimeters	**SLE**	systemic lupus erythematosus
d	day	**mmHg**	millimeters of mercury	**SOB**	shortness of breath
DDAVP	a medication used to treat hypoglycemia	**mo**	month	**sp. gr.**	specific gravity
				SQ	subcutaneous
DKA	diabetic ketoacidosis	**Na**	sodium	**s/s**	signs and symptoms
		ND	nursing diagnosis		
ECG	electrocardiogram/graph	**NG**	nasogastric	**tid**	three times daily
EEG	electroencephalograph	**NPO**	nothing by mouth	**TPN**	total parenteral nutrition
ET	endotracheal				
ETT	endotracheal tube	**O₂**	oxygen	**U/L**	units/liter
		OG	orogastric	**URI**	upper respiratory infection
F	fahrenheit	**O₂ sat(s)**	oxygen saturation value(s)		
FiO₂	fraction of inspired oxygen	**OT**	occupational therapy	**VS**	vital signs
FOB	foot of bed	**oz**	ounce		
FTT	failure to thrive			**WBC**	white blood cells
FUO	fever of undetermined origin	**PA**	pulmonary artery	**WNL**	within normal limits
		PaCO₂	partial arterial pressure, carbon dioxide	**yr**	year
g	gram				
GI	gastrointestinal	**PaO₂**	partial arterial pressure, oxygen	**x**	times, frequency

APPENDIX B: NORMAL VALUES

This appendix is organized in the way that test results are commonly grouped by laboratories.

SERUM ELECTROLYTES	DIFFERENTIAL BLOOD COUNT	STOOL	BLOOD GASES
SERUM CHEMISTRIES	URINE VALUES	OTHER	VITAL SIGNS
COMPLETE BLOOD COUNT (CBC)	CEREBROSPINAL FLUID	SWEAT	

SERUM ELECTROLYTES

TEST	SPECIMEN	AGE	RANGE
Chloride (Cl)	Serum	Newborn	97-110 mmol/L
		Thereafter	98-106 mmol/L
Potassium (K)	Serum	< 2 yr	3.0-6.0 mmol/L
		2-12 yr	3.5-7.0 mmol/L
		> 12 yr	3.5-5.0 mmol/L
Sodium (Na)	Serum	Newborn	134-146 mmol/L
		Infant	139-146 mmol/L
		Child	138-145 mmol/L
		Thereafter	136-146 mmol/L

SERUM CHEMISTRIES

TEST	SPECIMEN		AGE		RANGE
Bicarbonate	Serum				
		Arterial	Newborn/Child		21-28 mmol/L
		Venous	Newborn/Child		22-29 mmol/L
Bilirubin	Serum				
Total	Cord blood				< 2.0 mg/dL
	Serum		0-1 d		< 6.0 mg/dL
			1-2 d		< 8.0 mg/dL
			2-5 d		< 12.0 mg/dL
			> 5 d		2-1.0 mg/dL
Conjugated	Serum				0-0.2 mg/dL
Calcium, ionized (Ca)					
	Serum		Newborn	3-24 h	4.3-5.1 mg/dL
				24-48 h	4.0-4.7mg/dl
			Thereafter		4.8-4.92 mg/dL
			or		2.24-2.46 mEq/L
Calcium, total	Serum		Newborn	3-24 h	9.0-10.6 mg/dL
				24-48 h	7.0-12.0 mg/dL
				4-7 d	9.0-10.9 mg/dL
			Child		8.8-10.8 mg/dL
			Thereafter		8.4-10.2 mg/dL
Creatinine	Serum		Newborn		0.3-1.0 mg/dL
			Infant		0.2-0.4 mg/dL
			Child		0.3-0.7 mg/dL
			Adolescent		0.5-1.0 mg/dL
Creatinine Clearance (endogenous)	Serum		Newborn		40-65 mL/min/1.73 m^2
			< 40 yr		
				M	97-137 mL/min/1.73 m^2
				F	88-128 mL/min/1.73 m^2
			Decreases		6.5 mL/min/decade

Glucose	Serum	Newborn	1 d	40-60 mg/dL
			> 1 d	50-90 mg/dL
Glucose Tolerance Test		Child		60-100 mg/dL
		Adult		70-105 mg/dL
Glucose, 2 h pc	Serum	< 120 mg/dL (For diabetes, see Glucose Tolerance Test, oral)		
Magnesium	Plasma	0-6 d		1.2-2.6 mg/dL
		7d-2 yr		1.6-2.6 mg/dL
		2-14 yr		1.5-2.3 mg/dL
Protein, Total	Serum	Newborn		4.6-7.4 g/dL
		1-7 yr		6.1-7.9 g/dL
		8-12 yr		6.4-8.1 g/dL
		13-19 yr		6.6-8.2 g/dL

COMPLETE BLOOD COUNT (CBC)

TEST	SPECIMEN	AGE		RANGE
Erythrocyte count (RBC count)	Whole blood			Millions of cells/mm^3
		1-3 d (capillary)		4.0-6.6
		1 mo		3.0-5.4
		0.5-2 yr		3.7-5.3
		6-12 yr		4.0-5.2
		12-18 yr		
			M	4.5-5.3
			F	4.1-5.1
Erythrocyte Sedimentation Rate (ESR)	Whole blood	Child		0-10 mm/h
Hb	Whole blood	1-3 d (capillary)		14.5-22.5 g/dL
		2 mo		9.0-14.0 g/dL
		6-12 yr		11.5-15.5 g/dL
		12-18 yr		
			M	13.0-16.0 g/dL
			F	12.0-16.0 g/dL
Hct Percent PRBC (V Red Cells/V Whole Blood Cells x 100)	Whole blood	1 d (capillary)		48-69%
		2 mo		28-42%
		6-12 yr		35-45%
		12-18 yr		
			M	37-49%
			F	36-46%
Platelet count (thrombocyte count)	Whole blood	Newborn (same as adult after 1 week)		84-478x10^3/mm^3
		Adult		150-400 x 10^3/mm^3 (%L)

Reticulocyte count	Whole blood	1 d	0.4-0.6%
		7 d	< 0.1-1.3%
		1-4 week	< 1.0-1.2%
		5-6 week	< 0.1-2.4%
		7-8 week	0.1-2.9%
		9-10 week	< 0.1-2.6%
		11-12 week	0.1-1.3%
		Adult	0.5-1.5%

DIFFERENTIAL BLOOD COUNT

TEST	SPECIMEN	AGE	RANGE
Leukocyte differential	Whole blood	All Ages	
myelocytes			0
neutrophils—"bands"			3-5% – 150-400 cells/mm^3 (μL)
neutrophils—"segs"			54-62% – 3000-5800 cells/mm^3 (μL)
lymphocytes			25-33% – 1500-3000 cells/mm^3 (μL)
monocytes			3-7% – 285-500 cells/mm^3 (μL)
eosinophils			1-3% – 50-250 cells/mm^3 (μL)
basophils			0-0.75% – 15-50 cells/mm^3 (μL)

URINE VALUES

TEST	SPECIMEN	AGE	RANGE
Albumin	Urine	4-16 yr	3.35-15.3 mg/24h per 1.73 m^2
Bilirubin	Urine	All ages	negative
Creatinine	Urine	Full-term	10.4-19.7 mg/kg per 24h
		1.5-7 yr	10-15 mg/kg per 24h
		7-15 yr	5.2-41 mg/kg per 24h
Glucose		All ages	negative
Occult blood	Urine	All ages	negative
pH	Urine	Newborn/neonate	5-7
		Thereafter (average 6)	4.5-8
		All ages	negative
Sp. Gr.	Urine	Adult	1.002-1.030
		After 12-h fluid restriction	> 1.025
	Urine - 24 h specimen		1.015-1.025

Sediment:	Casts	Urine		All ages		
			Hyaline			seen occasionally (0-1)
			RBC			Not seen
			WBC			Not seen
	Cells	Urine		All ages		
			RBC			0-2/hpf
			WBC			
					M	0-3/hpf
					F	0-5/hpf
		Epithelial (more frequent in newborn)				Few
		Bacterial				No organisms
		Field Spun				< 20 organisms per hpf
Volume		Urine		Newborn		50-300 mL/24h
				Infant		350-550 mL/24h
				Child		500-1000 mL/24h
				Adolescent		700-1400 mL/24h (varies with intake and other factors)

CEREBROSPINAL FLUID

TEST	SPECIMEN	AGE	RANGE
Cell count	CSF	Newborn	0-20 mononuclear cells per mL
			0-10 polymorphonuclear cells per mL
			0-800 RBC per mL
		Neonate	0-5 mononuclear cells per mL
			0-10 polymorphonuclear cells per mL
			0-50 RBC per mL
		Thereafter	0-5 mononuclear cells per mL
Pressure	CSF		70-180 mm of water
Protein			
Total protein	CSF	All ages	8-32 mg/dL

STOOL

TEST	SPECIMEN	AGE		RANGE
Fat	Feces	Infant, breast-fed		< 1 g per 24h
		0-6 yr		< 2 g per 24h
		Adult		
			Normal diet	< 7 g per 24h
			Fat-free diet	< 4 g per 24h
Occult blood	Feces			Negative (< 2 mL blood per 24h in 100-200 g stool)

OTHER

TEST	SPECIMEN	AGE	RANGE	
Albumin	Plasma	Full term < 6 d	2.5-3.4 g/dL	
		< 5 yr	3.9-5.0 g/dL	
		5-19 yr	4.0-5.3 g/dL	
Amylase	Serum	1-19 yr	35-127 U/L	
Pancreatic isoenzymes	Serum	Cord blood - 8 mo	0-34%	
		9 mo-4 yr	5-56%	
		5-19 yr	23-59%	
Glucose Tolerance Test (GTT)	Oral Serum	All ages	Normal	Diabetic
Adult dose: 75 g	Fasting	All ages	70-105 mg/dL	> 115 mg/dL
Child dose: 1.75 g/kg of ideal	60 min	All ages	120-170 mg/dL	200 mg/dL
weight up to maximum of 75 g	90 min			
	120 min	All ages	100-140 mg/dL	200 mg/dL
			70-120 mg/dL	140 mg/dL
Phosphatase, alkaline	Serum	1-9 yr	145-200 U/L	
		10-11 yr	130-560 U/L	
			M	F
		12-13 yr	200-495 U/L	150-420 U/L
		14-15 yr	130-525 U/L	70-230 U/L
		16-19 yr	65-260 U/L	50-130 U/L
Thyroxine				
Free (FT)	Serum	Cord	8-13 µg/dL	
Total (T)	Serum	Newborn (lower in low-birth-weight infants)	11.5-24 µg/dL	
		Neonate	9-18 µg/dL	
		Infant	7-15 µg/dL	
		1-5 yr	7.3-15 µg/dL	
		5-10 yr	6.4-13.3 µg/dL	
		Thereafter	5-12 µg/dL	

SWEAT

TEST	SPECIMEN	AGE	RANGE
Chloride	Sweat	Normal	< 40 mmol/L
		Borderline	45-60 mmol/L
		Cystic fibrosis	> 60 mmol/L
Sodium	Sweat	Normal	< 40 mmol/L
		Indeterminate	45-60 mmol/L
		Cystic fibrosis	> 60 mmol/L

BLOOD GASES

TEST	SPECIMEN		AGE	RANGE
Base excess	Whole blood		Infant	(-2)-(+2) mmol/L
			Child	(-4)-(+2) mmol/L
			Thereafter	(-3)-(+3) mmol/L
Bicarbonate	Serum			
		Arterial	All ages	21-28 mmol/L
		Venous	All ages	22-29 mmol/L
PCO_2	Whole blood (arterial)		Newborn	27-40 mmHg
			Infant	27-41 mmHg
			Thereafter	
			M	35-48 mmHg
			F	32-45 mmHg
pH	Whole blood (arterial)		Full term birth	7.11-7.36
			1 d	7.29-7.45 ·
			Thereafter	7.35-7.45
PO_2	Whole blood (arterial)		> 1 h of age	55-80 mmHg
			1 d	54-95 mmHg
			Thereafter (decreases with age)	83-108 mmHg
SaO_2	Whole blood (arterial)		Newborn	85-90%
			Thereafter	95-99%

VITAL SIGNS

AVERAGE HEART RATE FOR CHILDREN AT REST

AGE	AVERAGE RATE		2 SD
Birth	140		50
1-6 mo	130		45
6-12 mo	115		40
1-2 yr	110		40
2-4 yr	105		35
6-10 yr	95		30
	M	F	
10-14 yr	65	85	30
14-18 yr	55	70	25

VARIATIONS IN RESPIRATION WITH AGE*

AGE	RATE/MIN
Premature	40-90
Neonate	30-80
1 yr	20-40
2-6 yr	20-30
6-10 yr	18-24
Adolescent	15-24

* These represent mean figures from several sources for both sexes. Vital capacity for boys averages about 6% greater than for girls.

AVERAGE NORMAL BLOOD PRESSURE FOR VARIOUS AGES (mmHg)*

AGE	SYSTOLIC	DIASTOLIC
1 d	78	42
1 mo	86	54
6 mo	90	60
1 yr	96	65
2-4 yr	99	65
6 yr	100	60
8 yr	105	60
10 yr	110	60
12 yr	115	60
14 yr	118	60
16 yr	120	65

* The figures for infants represent averages by the flush method.
NOTE: The figures under 1 year were obtained by the Doppler method. From 1 year on, the figures were obtained by auscultation, using the first change in sound to indicate diastolic pressure.

APPENDIX C: DEFINITIONS, CARE PLAN TOPICS

GENERAL

Chemotherapy: A systemic cancer treatment using drugs that affect the cell cycle; useful when there is disseminated disease or when there is a high risk of recurrence; can be curative, can prolong life, or can be palliative; is often used as an adjunct to surgery and/or radiation therapy.

Education for Discharge: Teaching the parent/child to perform care after discharge; various situations are addressed in the subsections of this care plan.

Grief: A natural human response to any loss, whether the loss is real, perceived, threatened, or anticipated.

Pain Management: Nursing interventions which are designed to prevent, reduce, or ameliorate pain and discomfort.

Radiation Therapy: Treatment of neoplastic disease by use of gamma rays to disturb proliferation of cells by decreasing the rate of mitosis or impairing DNA synthesis, thereby reducing tumor mass..

Postoperative Care: General nursing care for child following surgical intervention.

Postoperative Care, Infant: General nursing care for infant following surgical intervention

Preoperative Care: General nursing care that prepares the child and family for surgery.

Preoperative Care, Infant: General nursing care that prepares infant and family for surgery.

MEDICAL

Abuse, Neglect: Physical and/or psychological abuse/neglect including physical abuse, sexual abuse, and/or failure to thrive.

Aplastic Anemia: Anemia resulting from destruction of or injury to bone marrow stem cells or bone marrow matrix; exposure to toxins, specifically large doses of radiation, benzene, metabolites, alkylating agents, chloramphenicol, or sulfonamides. May cause pancytopenia.

Asthma, Bronchiolitis: An acute inflammation and spasm of smooth muscles in the bronchi and bronchioles, with increased mucus production and plugging; allergic hypersensitivity is most frequently caused by foreign substances, although infection, physical or psychological stress may trigger a response.

Autonomic Dysreflexia (Hyperreflexia): A sympathetic response characterized by paroxysmal hypertension leading to bradycardia, headache, flushing, and profuse sweating. It is usually due to visceral stimulation, i.e., UTI, impacted bowel, bladder distention, abdominal distention.

Biliary Atresia: Complete obstruction of the bile flow due to fibrosis or absence of the extrahepatic ducts.

Botulism: Ingestion of *Clostridium botulinum* (found in some sources of honey) leading to release of potentially lethal toxins in the bowel.

Brain Tumor: Abnormal growth(s) within the brain or its supporting structures of primary, metastatic, or developmental origin.

Cancer: Growth of abnormal cells that leads to destruction of healthy tissue and can ultimately lead to death.

Cerebral Palsy: A non-progressive, chronic disability, characterized by aberrant control of movement and posture, and appearing in early life.

Chemical Addiction/Withdrawal, Infant: The result of intrauterine exposure to drugs/chemicals taken by the mother; delivery cuts off the supply of these drugs and withdrawal behaviors are manifested.

Chemical Dependency, Adolescents: Intermittent or chronic use of stimulants or depressants resulting in alterations in mental and physiological function.

Chronic Lung Disease (Bronchopulmonary Dysplasia): Chronic lung condition with obstructive bronchiolitis, hyperinfiltration, and pulmonary fibrosis secondary to treatment for respiratory distress syndrome, including high oxygen concentrations delivered by positive pressure ventilation.

Cleft Lip, Cleft Palate: A congenital malformation of the lip and/or palate; surgical repair usually occurs within the first two years of life.

Congestive Heart Failure: A state in which the cardiac output is inadequate to meet the body's metabolic needs.

Crohn's Disease: Chronic, recurrent nonspecific inflammation of the entire intestine involving the mucosa and surrounding musculature and leading to deep fissure formation. Diarrhea, cramping, and malabsorption may occur.

Croup: An acute viral infection of the large airway (larynx, trachea, bronchi), which results in varying degrees of respiratory tract obstruction.

Cystic Fibrosis: An autosomal recessive disease; generalized dysfunction of exocrine glands occurs; production of thick mucus occurs, causing obstruction in several organs, most commonly the lungs, sweat glands, pancreas, liver, intestines, and reproductive tract.

Diabetic Ketoacidosis: Insulin deficiency, a life-threatening condition, occurs with the breakdown of fat (glycogenolysis) with ketones as a by-product; symptoms include dehydration, fruity-smelling breath, moderate to large ketones in urine, altered level of consciousness, difficulty with breathing. It is characterized by hyperglycemia, metabolic acidosis, increased plasma ketones and severe dehydration.

Diabetes Mellitus: A chronic disorder characterized by disturbances in carbohydrate, protein, and fat metabolism as a result of insufficient insulin. Two major classifications are type I, insulin-dependent diabetes mellitus, and type II, non-insulin-dependent diabetes mellitus.

Diarrhea, Dehydration: The frequent passage of loose, fluid, unformed stools leading to loss of essential fluids, causing dehydration.

315

Eating Disorders: Alterations in eating patterns due to physiologic and/or psychologic conditions.

Epiglottitis: A severe, rapidly progressing infection of the epiglottis and surrounding areas, resulting in inflammation and edema with the potential for a blocked airway.

Failure to Thrive: A child who is more than two standard deviations below the mean height and weight for age and sex, or fails to maintain a previously established growth pattern. Assessment for neglect and/or abuse is essential.

Fever of Undetermined Origin: Elevated temperature causing physiologic compromise with the underlying origin in question.

Gastroenteritis: A condition characterized by vomiting and diarrhea resulting from infection, allergy, intolerance of specific food substances, or ingestion of toxins.

Gastroesophageal Reflux: Spontaneous passage of acidic gastric contents from the stomach into the esophagus placing the child at risk for aspiration.

Guillain-Barré Syndrome: A neurological syndrome of acute ascending paralysis. Etiology is unknown, but syndrome generally follows a recent infection. Onset is rapid and symptoms are generally reversible.

Head Trauma: An open or closed injury to the cranium which places the child at risk for brain damage.

Hemophilia: An inherited coagulation abnormality caused by factor VIII deficiency. The abnormality is an X-linked trait.

Hepatitis: *Infectious Virus A (HAV)* - rapid onset of symptoms and destruction of liver cells caused by contaminated water or food. It usually affects young adults. *Serum Virus B (HBV)* - slow onset of symptoms and destruction of liver cells caused by contaminated serum from needles and instruments. It affects all age groups. *Non-A, Non-B, Hepatitis C* - little is known about this virus, but it manifests symptoms similar to HBV.

HIV/AIDS: Acquired Immune Deficiency Syndrome includes the final stages of a wide range of health problems caused by the human immunodeficiency virus type I (HIV) which attacks the cell-mediated immune system by invasion of T4 lymphocytes, placing the infected person at risk for opportunistic infections and cancers.

Hyperbilirubinemia: Elevation of unconjugated serum bilirubin concentration as evidenced by jaundice. It is caused by hemolytic disorders, infection, enzymatic deficiencies, maternal ingestion of sulfonamides or salicylates, or polycythemia.

Hypertension: Elevation of blood pressure.

Idiopathic Thrombocytic Purpura: A destruction of platelets caused by antibodies that are directed at platelet antigen.

Infectious Disorders: Disorders which can be transmitted through direct or indirect contact with infected person via a bacterial or viral agent.

Intracranial Pressure, Increased: Slow or sudden elevation in CSF pressure caused by edema, hemorrhage, trauma, or obstruction to outflow.

Juvenile Rheumatoid Arthritis: A chronic systemic autoimmune disease of unknown etiology characterized by an inflammatory reaction in the synovial membrane leading to destruction of joint cartilage and subsequent deformities.

Leukemia: A disease characterized by uncontrolled proliferation of leukocyte precursors in blood, marrow, and reticuloendothelial tissues.

Meningitis: Inflammation of the meninges, usually caused by an infectious agent, bacterial viral, tubercular, or mycotic.

Meningomyelocele, Repaired (older child): A congenital defect in the spinal vertebrae resulting in motor and sensory dysfunction of the trunk and lower extremities below the level of deformity and accompanied by nonfunctional bowel and bladder sphincters. Malformed cord

and roots are contained in a sac and covered by a thin vascular membrane.

Near-SIDS Event: Prolonged apneic event (usually nocturnal) that is identified by respiratory monitoring which prevents "unexpected" death in an at-risk population, i.e., premature male infants, infants of narcotic addicts, or children of smokers.

Nephrotic Syndrome: A syndrome resulting from degenerative changes in the kidneys without inflammation.

Neuroblastoma: A neural tumor; the second most common neoplasm in children.

Osteomyelitis: Infection of the long bones caused by acute local infection or bone trauma, usually caused by *Escherichia coli*, *Staphylococcus aureus*, or *Streptococcus pyogenes*.

Pneumonia: An inflammatory process of the lungs classified by area involved and/or causative agent.

Poisoning: The ingestion or accidental administration of a toxic dose of heavy metals, pharmacologics, or other materials or food.

Quadriplegia, Spinal Cord Injury: Paralysis of the upper and lower extremities resulting from injury to the spinal cord (thoracic and cervical regions).

Respiratory Distress Syndrome: Condition of decreased pulmonary gas exchange producing retention of carbon dioxide, usually resulting from deficiency of surfactant in immature lungs.

Reye Syndrome: An acute and life-threatening, multi-system disorder that follows a mild viral infection; seems to occur in association with aspirin intake during a viral illness.

Seizure Disorders: Sudden and violent involuntary motor movements of a group of skeletal muscles; generally are transitory and often involve disturbances in consciousness, motor-sensory, and/or autonomic functions.

Sickle Cell Disease: A genetic disease that occurs in individuals with a defective hemoglobin molecule (HbS); this defect results in a major rearrangement and rigid elongated, crescent-shaped, or sickle-shaped cells; oxygen tension is decreased, causing a shortened life span.

Systemic Lupus Erythematosus: A chronic, autoimmune inflammatory disease of the connective tissues that produces biochemical and structural changes in skin, joints, and muscles, usually with multiple organ involvement. The number of organs involved makes the disease an imitator of many other diagnoses.

Tuberculosis: A chronic acute or subacute infectious disease caused by the tubercle bacillus, mycobacterium tuberculosis, most commonly affecting the alveolar structure of the lung. Clinical presentation varies from asymptomatic, with only a positive skin test, to extensive pulmonary and systemic involvement.

Ulcerative Colitis: Inflammatory intestinal disease of unknown cause, usually affecting the mucosal lining of the colon; may be mild, chronic, or acute.

Wilms' Tumor (nephroblastoma): A malignant neoplasm of the kidney; most often occuring in young children.

SURGICAL

Appendectomy: Procedure to remove an obstruction of the appendiceal lumen progressively causing inflammation, distention, decreased blood supply, necrosis, and perforation of the appendix. Perforation causes generalized peritonitis or a localized abscess.

Burns and Grafts: *Superficial* - epidermis is red, with no blister formation. *Partial thickness* - epidermal and dermal layers are blistered with subcutaneous edema and pain. *Full thickness* - all layers of skin are involved and fat, muscle, nerves, blood supply, and bone may be affected.

Grafts: The surgical placement of skin to reestablish skin integrity in wounds that cannot heal via processes of epithelialization and contraction.

Cardiac Surgery: Surgical procedures that provide palliative or restorative function of the heart and/or cardiovascular system.

Cleft Lip Repair and Cleft Palate Repair: Surgical repair of congenital interruption in the development of the upper lip and/or of the oral palate. Repair to lip may be unilateral or bilateral. Repair to palate may involve the hard or soft palate, or both.

Colon Surgery, Adolescent : Surgical opening into the intestine to provide temporary or permanent passage of feces, necessitated by inflammation, trauma, or obstruction.

Fundolplication: A surgical procedure used to minimize gastroesophageal reflux; proximal stomach is wrapped around the distal esophagus, crafting a junction which prevents reflux.

Gastrostomy: A surgically constructed stoma or opening for a catheter to the stomach when there is need for feedings, or decompressions and drainage.

Head Trauma, Surgical Management: Surgical relief or repair of trauma to the cranium. Also see *Head Trauma* in Medical Care Plans section.

Hirschsprung's Disease, Pull-Through: Surgical treatment of a congenital condition characterized by greatly dilated colon proximal to an area of narrowing, usually in the rectum or rectosigmoid, resulting from absence of parasympathetic ganglion cells and peristalsis.

Hypospadias Repair: Surgical repair of hypospadias, movement of meatal opening to the glans penis.

Mastoidectomy: Resection of inflamed mastoid bone, associated with chronic middle ear infection.

Neuroblastoma Repair: Surgical repair of a neuroblastoma, the second most common neoplasm in children. Also see *Neuroblastoma* in Medical Care Plans section.

Orthopedic Repair, Limb Fractures: Surgical repair of skeletal fractures.

Pyloric Stenosis Repair: Surgical repair of congenital obstruction of the gastric pylorus caused by hypertrophy of the circular pyloric musculature. Symptoms usually appear in the second or third week of life; occurring most frequently in males.

Renal Surgery: Surgical intervention to ameliorate a kidney disorder or associated condition.

Tracheostomy: Insertion of a tube into the trachea through a surgical incision to facilitate an airway.

Ventricular Shunt Revision: A treatment for noncommunicating hydrocephalus involving surgical placement of device that bypasses cranial obstruction and carries CSF to an extracranial site where fluid is then absorbed.

APPENDIX D: NANDA NURSING DIAGNOSES

This list represents the NANDA nursing diagnoses approved for clinical use and testing (1992).

Pattern 1: Exchanging

1.1.2.1.*	Altered ⁺**Nutrition**: More than body requirements
1.1.2.2.	Altered **Nutrition**: Less than body requirements
1.1.2.3.	Altered **Nutrition**: Potential for more than body requirements
1.2.1.1.	High Risk for **Infection**
1.2.2.1.	High Risk for Altered **Body Temperature**
1.2.2.2.	Hypothermia
1.2.2.3.	Hyperthermia
1.2.2.4.	Ineffective **Thermoregulation**
1.2.3.1.	**Dysreflexia**
1.3.1.1.	**Constipation**
1.3.1.1.1.	Perceived **Constipation**
1.3.1.1.2.	Colonic **Constipation**
1.3.1.2.	**Diarrhea**
1.3.1.3.	**Bowel** Incontinence
1.3.2.	Altered **Urinary** Elimination
1.3.2.1.1.	Stress Incontinence **(Urinary)**
1.3.2.1.2.	Reflex Incontinence **(Urinary)**
1.3.2.1.3.	Urge Incontinence **(Urinary)**
1.3.2.1.4.	Functional Incontinence **(Urinary)**
1.3.2.1.5.	Total Incontinence **(Urinary)**
1.3.2.2.	**Urinary** Retention
1.4.1.1.	Altered **Tissue Perfusion** (Specify Type) (Renal, cerebral, cardiopulmonary, gastrointestinal, peripheral)
1.4.1.2.1.	**Fluid** Volume Excess
1.4.1.2.2.1.	**Fluid** Volume Deficit
1.4.1.2.2.2.	High Risk for **Fluid** Volume Deficit
1.4.2.1.	Decreased **Cardiac** Output
1.5.1.1.	Impaired **Gas** Exchange
1.5.1.2.	Ineffective **Airway** Clearance
1.5.1.3.1.	Inability to Sustain Spontaneous **Ventilation**
1.5.1.3.2.	Dysfunctional **Ventilatory** Weaning Response (DVWR)
1.6.1.	High Risk for **Injury**
1.6.1.1.	High Risk for **Suffocation**
1.6.1.2.	High Risk for **Poisoning**
1.6.1.3.	High Risk for **Trauma**
1.6.1.4.	High Risk for **Aspiration**
1.6.1.5	High Risk for **Disuse Syndrome**
1.6.2.	Altered **Protection**
1.6.2.1.	Impaired **Tissue Integrity**
1.6.2.1.1.	Altered **Oral** Mucous Membrane
1.6.2.1.2.1.	Impaired **Skin** Integrity
1.6.2.1.2.2.	High Risk for Impaired **Skin** Integrity

Pattern 2: Communicating

2.1.1.1.	Impaired Verbal **Communication**

Pattern 3: Relating

3.1.1.	Impaired **Social Interaction**
3.1.2.	**Social Isolation**
3.2.1.	Altered **Role** Performance
3.2.1.1.1.	Altered **Parenting**
3.2.1.1.2.	High Risk for Altered **Parenting**
3.2.1.2.1.	**Sexual** Dysfunction
3.2.2.	Altered **Family** Processes
3.2.2.1.	**Caregiver** Role Strain
3.2.2.2.	High Risk for **Caregiver** Role Strain
3.2.3.1.	**Parental** Role Conflict
3.3.	Altered **Sexuality** Patterns

Pattern 4: Valuing

4.1.1.	**Spiritual Distress** (Distress of the Human Spirit)

Pattern 5: Choosing

5.1.1.1.	Ineffective Individual **Coping**
5.1.1.1.1.	Impaired **Adjustment**
5.1.1.1.2.	Defensive **Coping**
5.1.1.1.3.	Ineffective **Denial**
5.1.2.1.1.	Ineffective Family **Coping**: Disabling
5.1.2.1.2.	Ineffective Family **Coping**: Compromised
5.1.2.2.	Family **Coping**: Potential for growth
5.2.1.	Ineffective Management of **Therapeutic** Regimen (Individuals)
5.2.1.1.	**Noncompliance** (Specify)
5.3.1.1	**Decisional** Conflict (Specify)
5.4.	**Health** Seeking Behaviors (Specify)

Pattern 6: Moving

6.1.1.1.	Impaired Physical **Mobility**
6.1.1.1.1.	High Risk for **Peripheral Neurovascular** Dysfunction
6.1.1.2.	**Activity** Intolerance
6.1.1.2.1.	**Fatigue**
6.1.1.3.	High Risk for **Activity** Intolerance
6.2.1.	**Sleep** Pattern Disturbance
6.3.1.1.	**Diversional** Activity Deficit
6.4.1.1.	Impaired **Home Maintenance** Management
6.4.2.	Altered **Health Maintenance**
6.5.1.	Feeding **Self-Care Deficit**
6.5.1.1.	Impaired **Swallowing**
6.5.1.2.	Ineffective **Breastfeeding**
6.5.1.2.1.	Interrupted **Breastfeeding**
6.5.1.3.	Effective **Breastfeeding**
6.5.1.4.	Ineffective **Infant** Feeding Pattern
6.5.2.	Bathing/Hygiene **Self-Care Deficit**
6.5.3.	Dressing/Grooming **Self-Care Deficit**
6.5.4.	Toileting **Self-Care Deficit**
6.6.	Altered **Growth** and Development
6.7.	**Relocation** Stress Syndrome

Pattern 7: Perceiving

7.1.1.	**Body Image** Disturbance
7.1.2.	**Self-Esteem** Disturbance
7.1.2.1.	Chronic Low **Self-Esteem**
7.1.2.2.	Situational Low **Self-Esteem**
7.1.3.	**Personal** Identity Disturbance
7.2.	**Sensory/Perceptual** Alterations (Specify): visual, auditory, kinesthetic, gustatory, tactile, olfactory
7.2.1.1.	**Unilateral** Neglect
7.3.1.	**Hopelessness**
7.3.2.	**Powerlessness**

Pattern 8: Knowing

8.1.1.	**Knowledge** Deficit (Specify)
8.3.	Altered **Thought** Processes
9.1.1.	**Pain**
9.1.1.1.	Chronic **Pain**
9.2.1.1.	Dysfunctional **Grieving**
9.2.1.2	Anticipatory **Grieving**
9.2.2.	High Risk for **Violence**: Self-directed or directed at others
9.2.2.1.	High Risk for **Self-Mutilation**
9.2.3.	**Post-Trauma** Response
9.2.3.1.	**Rape-Trauma** Syndrome
9.2.3.1.1.	**Rape-Trauma Syndrome**: Compound Reaction
9.2.3.1.2.	**Rape-Trauma Syndrome**: Silent Reaction
9.3.1.	**Anxiety**
9.3.2.	**Fear**

* Numbers refer to location in *NANDA Nursing Diagnoses: Definitions and Classifications 1992-1993*.

⁺ Bold type indicates alphabetical location in Appendix E.

This appendix includes only the definitions and defining characteristics of those nursing diagnoses that are used in this book.
Abridged from NANDA Nursing Diagnoses: Definitions and Classification, 1992

ACTIVITY INTOLERANCE A state in which an individual has insufficient physiological or psychological energy to endure or complete required or desired daily activities. **Defining Characteristics:** Verbal report of fatigue or weakness; abnormal heart rate or blood pressure response to activity; exertional discomfort or dyspnea; electrocardiographic changes reflecting arrhythmias or ischemia.

ACTIVITY INTOLERANCE: HIGH RISK FOR A state in which an individual is at risk of experiencing insufficient physiological or psychological energy to endure or complete required or desired daily activities. **Defining Characteristics:** *Presence of risk factors such as:* History of previous intolerance; deconditioned status; presence of circulatory/respiratory problems; inexperience with the activity.

AIRWAY CLEARANCE, INEFFECTIVE A state in which an individual is unable to clear secretions or obstructions from the respiratory tract to maintain airway patency. **Defining Characteristics:** Abnormal breath sounds (rales [crackles], rhonchi [wheezes]); changes in rate or depth of respiration; tachypnea; cough, effective/ineffective, with or without sputum, cyanosis; dyspnea.

ANXIETY A vague uneasy feeling whose source is often nonspecific or unknown to the individual. **Defining Characteristics:** *Subjective:* Increased tension; apprehension; painful and persistent increased helplessness; uncertainty; fearful; scared; regretful; overexcited; rattled; distressed; jittery; feelings of inadequacy; shakiness; fear of unspecific consequences; expressed concerns regarding change in life events; worried; anxious. *Objective:* Sympathetic stimulation-cardiovascular excitation, superficial vasoconstriction, pupil dilation; restlessness; insomnia; glancing about; poor eye contact; trembling/hand tremors; extraneous movement (foot shuffling, hand/arm movements); facial tension; voice quivering; focus "self"; increased wariness; increased perspiration.

ASPIRATION: HIGH RISK FOR The state in which an individual is at risk for entry of gastrointestinal secretions, oropharyngeal secretions, solids or fluids into tracheo-bronchial passages. **Defining Characteristics:** *Presence of risk factors such as:* Reduced level of consciousness; depressed cough and gag reflexes; presence of tracheostomy or endotracheal tube; incomplete lower esophageal sphincter; gastrointestinal tubes; tube feedings; medication administration; situations hindering elevation of upper body; increased intragastric pressure; increased gastric residual; decreased gastrointestinal motility; delayed gastric emptying; impaired swallowing; facial/oral/neck surgery or trauma; wired jaws.

BODY IMAGE DISTURBANCE Disruption in the way one perceives one's body image. **Defining Characteristics:** A or B must be present to justify the diagnosis of Body Image Disturbance. **A =** verbal response to actual or perceived change in structure and/or function. **B =** non-verbal response to actual or perceived change in structure and/or function. The following clinical manifestations may be used to validate the presence of A or B. *Objective:* Missing body part; actual change in structure and/or function; not looking at body part; not touching body part; hiding or overexposing body part (intentional or unintentional); trauma to nonfunctioning part; change in social involvement; change in ability to estimate spatial relationship of body to environment. *Subjective:* Verbalization of: change in lifestyle; fear of rejection or of reaction by others; focus on past strength, function, or appearance; negative feelings about body; feelings of helplessness, hopelessness, or powerlessness; preoccupations with change or loss; emphasis on remaining strengths, heightened achievement; extension of body boundary to incorporate environmental objects; personalization of part or loss by name; depersonalization of part or loss by impersonal pronouns; refusal to verify actual change.

BODY TEMPERATURE, ALTERED: HIGH RISK FOR The state in which the individual is at risk for failure to maintain body temperature within normal range. **Defining Characteristics:** *Presence of risk factors such as:* Extremes of age; extremes of weight; exposure to cold/cool or warm/hot environments; dehydration; inactivity or vigorous activity; medications causing vasoconstriction/vasodilation; altered metabolic rate; sedation; inappropriate clothing for environmental temperature; illness or trauma affecting temperature regulation.

BOWEL INCONTINENCE A state in which an individual experiences a change in normal bowel habits characterized by involuntary passage of stool.

BREATHING PATTERN, INEFFECTIVE The state in which an individual's inhalation and/or exhalation pattern does not enable adequate pulmonary inflation or emptying. **Defining Characteristics:** Dyspnea; shortness of breath; tachypnea; fremitus; abnormal arterial blood gas; cyanosis; cough; nasal flaring; respiratory depth changes; assumption of 3-point position; pursed-lip breathing/prolonged expiratory phase; increased anteroposterior diameter; use of accessory muscles; altered chest excursion.

CARDIAC OUTPUT, DECREASED A state in which the blood pumped by an individual's heart is sufficiently reduced that it is inadequate to meet the needs of the body's tissues. **Defining Characteristics:** Variations in blood pressure readings, arrhythmias; fatigue; jugular vein distention; color changes, skin and mucous membranes; oliguria; decreased peripheral pulses; cold clammy skin; rales; dyspnea, orthopnea; restlessness. **Other Possible Characteristics:** Change in mental status; shortness of breath; syncope; vertigo; edema; cough; frothy sputum; gallop rhythm; weakness.

COMMUNICATION, IMPAIRED: VERBAL The state in which an individual experiences a decreased or absent ability to use or understand language in human interaction. **Defining Characteristics:** Unable to speak dominant language; speaks or verbalizes with difficulty; does not or cannot speak; stuttering; slurring; difficulty forming words or sentences; difficulty expressing thought verbally; inappropriate verbalization; dyspnea; disorientation.

CONSTIPATION A state in which an individual experiences a change in normal bowel habits characterized by a decrease in frequency of stools and/or passage of hard, dry stools. **Defining Characteristics:** Decreased activity level; frequency less than usual pattern; hard, formed stools; palpable mass; reported feeling of pressure or fullness in rectum; straining at stool. **Other Possible Characteristics:** Abdominal pain; appetite impairment; back pain; headache; interference with daily living; use of laxatives.

CONSTIPATION, COLONIC The state in which an individual's pattern of elimination is characterized by hard, dry stool which results from a delay in passage of food residue. **Defining Characteristics:** *Major:* Decreased frequency; hard, dry stool; straining at stool; painful defecation; abdominal distention; palpable mass. *Minor:* Rectal pressure; headache; appetite impairment; abdominal pain.

COPING, FAMILY: POTENTIAL FOR GROWTH Effective management of adaptive tasks by family member involved with the client's health challenge; family member exhibits desire and readiness for enhanced health and growth in regard to self and in relation to the client. **Defining Characteristics:** Family member attempts to describe growth impact of crisis on his or her own values, priorities, goals, or relationships; family member is moving in direction of lifestyle that supports and monitors health and the maturational processes; audits and negotiates treatment programs; generally chooses experiences that optimize wellness; individual expresses interest in making contact on a one-to-one basis or on a mutual-aid group basis with another person who has experienced a similar situation.

COPING, INEFFECTIVE FAMILY: COMPROMISED A usually supportive primary person (family member or close friend) provides insufficient, ineffective, or compromised support, comfort, assistance or encouragement which may be needed by the client to manage or master adaptive tasks related to his or her health challenge. **Defining Characteristics:** *Subjective:* Client expresses or confirms a

concern or complaint about significant other's response to his or her health problem; significant person describes preoccupation with personal reaction (fear, anticipatory grief, guilt, anxiety) to client's illness, disability, or other situational or developmental crises; significant person describes or confirms an inadequate understanding or knowledge base which interferes with effective assistance or supportive behaviors. *Objective:* Significant person attempts assistive or supportive behaviors with less than satisfactory results; significant person withdraws or enters into limited or temporary personal communication with the client at the time of need; significant person displays protective behavior disproportionate (too little or too much) to the client's abilities or need for autonomy.

COPING, INEFFECTIVE FAMILY: DISABLING Behavior of significant person (family member or other primary person) that disables his or her own capacities and the client's capacities to effectively address tasks essential to either person's adaptation to the health challenge. **Defining Characteristics:** Neglectful care of the client in regard to basic human needs and/or illness treatment; distortion of reality regarding the client's health problem, including extreme denial about its existence or severity; intolerance; rejection; abandonment; desertion; carrying on usual routines while disregarding client's needs; psychosomaticism; takes on illness signs of client; decisions and actions by family which are detrimental to economic or social well-being; agitation; depression; aggression, hostility; impaired restructuring of a meaningful life for self; impaired individualization; prolonged over-concern for client; neglectful relationships with other family members; client's development of helpless, inactive dependence.

COPING: INEFFECTIVE INDIVIDUAL Impairment of adaptive behaviors and problem-solving abilities of a person in meeting life's demands and roles. **Defining Characteristics:** Verbalization of inability to cope or inability to ask for help; inability to meet role expectations; inability to meet basic needs; inability to problem-solve; alteration in societal participation; destructive behavior toward self or others; inappropriate use of defense mechanisms; change in usual

communication patterns; verbal manipulation; high illness rate; high rate of accidents.

DIARRHEA A state in which an individual experiences a change in normal bowel habits characterized by the frequent passage of loose, fluid, unformed stools. **Defining Characteristics:** Abdominal pain; cramping; increased frequency; increased frequency of bowel sounds; loose, liquid stools; urgency. **Other Possible Characteristics:** Change in color.

DIVERSIONAL ACTIVITY DEFICIT The state in which an individual experiences a decreased stimulation from or interest in or engagement in recreational or leisure activities. **Defining Characteristics:** Patient makes statements regarding boredom, wishes there was something to do or something to read, etc.; usual hobbies cannot be undertaken in hospital.

FAMILY PROCESSES, ALTERED The state in which a family that normally functions effectively experiences a dysfunction. **Defining Characteristics:** Family system unable to meet physical needs of its members; family system unable to meet emotional, security, or spiritual needs of its members; parents do not demonstrate respect for each other's views on childrearing practices; inability to express/accept wide range of feelings; inability to express/accept feelings of members; inability of the family members to relate to each other for mutual growth and maturation; family uninvolved in community activities; inability to accept/receive help appropriately; rigidity in function and roles; family not demonstrating respect for individuality and autonomy of its members; family unable to adapt to change, deal with traumatic experience constructively; family failing to accomplish current/past developmental task; unhealthy family decision-making process; failure to send and receive clear messages; inappropriate boundary maintenance; inappropriate/poorly communicated family rules, rituals, symbols; unexamined family myths; inappropriate level and direction of energy.

FATIGUE An overwhelming sustained sense of exhaustion and decreased capacity for physical and mental work. **Defining Characteristics:** *Major:* Verbalization of an unremitting and/or overwhelming lack of energy; inability to maintain usual routines. *Minor:* Perceived need for additional energy to accomplish routine tasks; increase in physical complaints; emotionally labile or irritable; impaired ability to concentrate; decreased performance; lethargy or listlessness; disinterest in surroundings/introspection; decreased libido; accident proneness.

FEAR Feeling of dread related to an identifiable source which the person validates. **Defining Characteristics:** Ability to identify object of fear.

FLUID VOLUME DEFICIT The state in which an individual experiences vascular, cellular, or intracellular dehydration. **Defining Characteristics:** Change in urine output; change in urine concentration; sudden weight loss or gain; decreased venous filling; hemoconcentration; change in serum sodium. **Other Possible Characteristics:** Hypotension; thirst; increased pulse rate; decreased skin turgor; decreased pulse volume/pressure; change in mental state; increased body temperature; dry skin; dry mucous membranes; weakness.

FLUID VOLUME DEFICIT: HIGH RISK FOR The state in which an individual is at risk of experiencing vascular, cellular, or intracellular dehydration. **Defining Characteristics:** *Presence of risk factors such as:* Extremes of age; extremes of weight; excessive losses through normal routes, e.g., diarrhea; loss of fluid through abnormal routes, e.g., indwelling tubes; deviations affecting access to or intake or absorption of fluids, e.g., physical immobility; factors influencing fluid needs, e.g., hypermetabolic state; knowledge deficiency related to fluid volume; medications, e.g., diuretics.

FLUID VOLUME EXCESS The state in which an individual experiences increased fluid retention and edema. **Defining Characteristics:** Edema; effusion; anasarca; weight gain; shortness of breath, orthopnea; intake greater than output; S/3 heart sound; pulmonary congestion (chest x-ray); abnormal breath sounds, rales (crackles); change in respiratory pattern; change in mental status; decreased hemoglobin and hematocrit; blood pressure changes; central venous pressure changes;

pulmonary artery pressure changes; jugular vein distention; positive hepatojugular reflex; oliguria; specific gravity changes, azotemia, altered electrolytes; restlessness and anxiety.

GAS EXCHANGE, IMPAIRED The state in which the individual experiences a decreased passage of oxygen and/or carbon dioxide between the alveoli of the lungs and the vascular system. **Defining Characteristics:** Confusion; somnolence; restlessness; irritability; inability to move secretions; hypercapnea; hypoxia.

GRIEVING, ANTICIPATORY Potential loss of significant object; expression of distress at potential loss; denial of potential loss; guilt; anger; sorrow; choked feelings; changes in eating habits; alterations in sleep patterns; alterations in activity level; altered libido; altered communication patterns.

GROWTH AND DEVELOPMENT, ALTERED: The state in which an individual demonstrates deviations in norms from his/her age group. **Defining Characteristics:** *Major:* Delay or difficulty in performing skills (motor, social, or expressive) typical of age group; altered physical growth; inability to perform self-care or self-control activities appropriate for age. *Minor:* Flat affect; listlessness, decreased responses.

HEALTH MAINTENANCE, ALTERED Inability to identify, manage and/or seek out help to maintain health. **Defining Characteristics:** Demonstrated lack of knowledge regarding basic health practices; demonstrated lack of adaptive behaviors to internal/external environmental changes; reported or observed inability to take responsibility for meeting basic health practices in any or all functional pattern areas; history of lack of health-seeking behavior; expressed interest in improving health behaviors; reported or observed lack of equipment, financial and/or other resources; reported or observed impairment of personal support systems.

HYPERTHERMIA A state in which an individual's body temperature is elevated above his/her normal range. **Defining Characteristics:** *Major:* Increase in body temperature above normal range. *Minor:* Flushed skin, warm to touch; increased

respiratory rate; tachycardia; seizures/convulsions.

HYPOTHERMIA The state in which an individual's body temperature is reduced below normal range. **Defining Characteristics:** *Major:* Reduction in body temperature below normal range; shivering (mild); cool skin; pallor (moderate). *Minor:* Slow capillary refill; tachycardia; cyanotic nail beds; hypertension; piloerection.

INFECTION: HIGH RISK FOR The state in which an individual is at increased risk for being invaded by pathogenic organisms. **Defining Characteristics:** *Presence of risk factors such as:* Inadequate primary defenses (broken skin, traumatized tissue, decrease in ciliary action, stasis of body fluids, change in pH secretions, altered peristalsis); inadequate secondary defenses (e.g., decreased hemoglobin, leukopenia, suppressed inflammatory response) and immunosuppression; inadequate acquired immunity; tissue destruction and increased environmental exposure; chronic disease; invasive procedures; malnutrition; pharmaceutical agents; trauma; rupture of amniotic membranes; insufficient knowledge to avoid exposure to pathogens.

INJURY: HIGH RISK FOR A state in which the individual is at risk of injury as a result of environmental conditions interacting with the individual's adaptive and defensive resources. **Defining Characteristics:** *Presence of risk factors such as: Internal:* Biochemical, regulatory function (sensory dysfunction, integrative dysfunction, effector dysfunction, tissue hypoxia); malnutrition; autoimmune; abnormal blood profile (leukocytosis/leukopenia, altered clotting factors, thrombocytopenia, sickle cell, thalassemia, decreased hemoglobin); physical (broken skin, altered mobility); developmental age (physiological, psychosocial); psychological (affective, orientation). *External:* Biological (immunization level of community, microorganism); chemical (pollutants, poisons, drugs, pharmaceutical agents, alcohol, caffeine, nicotine, preservatives, cosmetics, and dyes); nutrients (vitamins, food types); physical (design, structure, and arrangement of community, building, and/or equipment); mode of transport/transportation; people/provider (nosocomial agents; staffing patterns;

cognitive, affective, and psychomotor factors).

KNOWLEDGE DEFICIT (SPECIFY)
Defining Characteristics: Verbalization of problem; inaccurate follow-through of instruction; inaccurate performance of test; inappropriate or exaggerated behaviors, e.g., hysterical, hostile, agitated, apathetic.

MOBILITY, IMPAIRED PHYSICAL A
state in which the individual experiences a limitation of ability* for independent physical movement. **Defining Characteristics:** Inability to purposefully move within the physical environment, including bed mobility, transfer, and ambulation; reluctance to attempt movement; limited range of motion; decreased muscle strength, control, and/or mass; imposed restrictions of movement, including mechanical, medical protocol; impaired coordination.

SUGGESTED FUNCTIONAL LEVEL CLASSIFICATION
0 = completely independent
1 = requires use of equipment or device
2 = requires help from another person, for assistance, supervision, or teaching
3 = requires help from another person and equipment device
4 = dependent, does not participate in activity.
Code adapted from E. Jones, et al. *Patient Classification for Long-Term Care: Users' Manual*, HEW, Publication No. HRA-74-3107, November 1974.

NUTRITION, ALTERED: LESS THAN BODY REQUIREMENTS The state in
which an individual experiences an intake of nutrients insufficient to meet metabolic needs. **Defining Characteristics:** Loss of weight with or without adequate food intake; reported inadequate food intake less than RDA (recommended daily allowance); weakness of muscles required for swallowing or mastication; body weight 20% or more under ideal; reported or evident lack of food; aversion to eating; lack of interest in food; reported altered taste sensation; satiety immediately after ingesting food; abdominal pain with or without pathology; sore, inflamed buccal cavity; capillary fragility; abdominal cramping; diarrhea and/or steatorrhea; hyperactive bowel sounds; perceived inability to ingest food; pale conjunctival and mucous membranes; poor muscle tone;

excessive loss of hair; lack of information, misinformation.

ORAL MUCOUS MEMBRANE, ALTERED The state in which an
individual experiences disruptions in the tissue layers of the oral cavity. **Defining Characteristics:** Oral pain/discomfort; coated tongue; xerostomia (dry mouth); stomatitis; oral lesions or ulcers; lack of or decreased salivation; leukoplakia; edema; hyperemia; oral plaque; desquamation; vesicles; hemorrhagic gingivitis, carious teeth; halitosis.

PAIN (Acute) A state in which an
individual experiences and reports the presence of severe discomfort or an uncomfortable sensation. **Defining Characteristics:** *Subjective:* Describes or communicates (verbal or coded) pain. *Objective:* Guarding behavior, protective; self-focusing; narrowed focus (altered time perception, withdrawal from social contact, impaired thought process); distraction behavior (moaning, crying, pacing, seeking out other people and/or activities, restlessness); facial mask of pain (eyes lack luster, "beaten look," fixed or scattered movement, grimace); alteration in muscle tone (may span from listless to rigid); autonomic responses not seen in chronic stable pain (diaphoresis, blood pressure and pulse change, pupillary dilation, increased or decreased respiratory rate).

PAIN, CHRONIC A state in which the
individual experiences pain that continues for more than six months in duration. **Defining Characteristics:** *Major:* Verbal report or observed evidence of pain experienced for more than six months. *Minor:* Fear of reinjury; physical and social withdrawal; altered ability to continue previous activities; anorexia; weight changes; changes in sleep patterns; facial mask; guarded movement.

PARENTAL ROLE CONFLICT The
state in which a parent experiences role confusion and conflict in response to crisis. **Defining Characteristics:** *Major:* Parent(s) express concerns/feelings of inadequacy to provide for child's physical and emotional needs during hospitalization or in the home; demonstrated disruption in caretaking routines; parent(s) express concerns about changes in parental role, family functioning, family communication, or family health. *Minor:* Express concern about perceived loss of control over

decisions relating to their child; reluctant to participate in usual caretaking activities even with encouragement and support; verbalize or demonstrate feelings of guilt, anger, fear, anxiety and/or frustrations about effect of child's illness on family process.

⁺PARENTING, ALTERED The state in
which a nurturing figure(s) experiences an inability to create an environment which promotes the optimum growth and development of another human being. **Defining Characteristics:** Abandonment; runaway; verbalizes lack of control of child; incidence of physical and psychological trauma; lack of parental attachment behaviors; inappropriate visual, tactile, auditory stimulation; negative identification of infant/child's characteristics; negative attachment of meanings to infant/child's characteristics; constant verbalization of disappointment in gender or physical characteristics of the infant/child; verbalization of resentment towards the infant/child; verbalization of role inadequacy; inattentive to infant/child needs; verbal disgust at body functions of infant/child; noncompliance with health appointments for self and/or infant/child; inappropriate caretaking behavior (toilet training, sleep/rest, feeding); inappropriate or inconsistent discipline practices; frequent accidents; frequent illness; growth and development lag in the child; history of child abuse or abandonment by primary caretaker; verbalizes desire to have child call him/herself by first name versus traditional cultural tendencies; child receives care from multiple caretakers without consideration for the needs of the infant/child; compulsively seeking role approval from others.

⁺PARENTING, ALTERED: HIGH RISK FOR The state in which a nurturing
figure(s) is at risk to experience an inability to create an environment which promotes the optimum growth and development of another human being. **Defining Characteristics:** *Presence of risk factors such as:* Lack of parental attachment behaviors; inappropriate visual, tactile, auditory stimulation; negative identification or attachment of meanings of infant/child's characteristics; constant verbalization of disappointment in gender or physical characteristics of the infant/child; verbalization of resentment towards the infant/child; verbalization of role inadequacy; inattentive to

infant/child's needs; verbal disgust at body functions of infant/child; noncompliance with health appointments for self and/or infant/child; inappropriate caretaking behaviors (toilet training, sleep/rest, feeding); inappropriate or inconsistent discipline practices; frequent accidents; frequent illness; growth and development lag in the child; history of child abuse or abandonment by primary caretaker; verbalizes desire to have child call him/herself by first name versus traditional cultural tendencies; child receives care from multiple caretakers without consideration for the needs of the infant/child; compulsively seeking role approval from others.

⁺It is important to state as a preface to parenting diagnoses that adjustment to parenting in general is a normal maturational process that elicits nursing behaviors of prevention of potential problems and health promotion.

POISONING: HIGH RISK FOR
Accentuated risk of accidental exposure to or ingestion of drugs or dangerous products in doses sufficient to cause poisoning. **Defining Characteristics:** *Presence of risk factors such as: Internal (individual):* Reduced vision; verbalization of occupational setting without adequate safeguards; lack of safety or drug education; lack of proper precaution; cognitive or emotional difficulties; insufficient finances. *External (environmental):* Large supplies of drugs in house; medicines stored in unlocked cabinets accessible to children or confused persons; dangerous products placed or stored within the reach of children or confused persons; availability of illicit drugs potentially contaminated by poisonous additives; flaking, peeling paint or plaster in presence of young children; chemical contamination of food and water; unprotected contact with heavy metals, chemicals, paint, lacquer, etc., in poorly ventilated areas or without effective protection; presence of poisonous vegetation; presence of atmospheric pollutants.

POWERLESSNESS Perception that one's own action will not significantly affect an outcome; a perceived lack of control over a current situation or immediate happening. *Defining Characteristics: Severe:* Verbal expressions of having no control or influence over

situation or its outcome; verbal expressions of having no control over self-care; depression over physical deterioration which occurs despite patient compliance with regimens; apathy. *Moderate:* Nonparticipation in care or decision-making when opportunities are provided; expressions of dissatisfaction and frustration over inability to perform previous tasks and/or activities; does not monitor progress; expression of doubt regarding role performance; reluctance to express true feelings; fearing alienation from caregivers; passivity; inability to seek information regarding care; dependence on others that may result in irritability, resentment, anger, and guilt; does not defend self-care practices when challenged. *Low:* Expressions of uncertainty about fluctuating energy levels; passivity.

PROTECTION, ALTERED The state in which an individual experiences a decrease in the ability to guard the self from internal or external threats such as illness or injury. **Defining Characteristics:** *Major:* Deficient immunity; impaired healing; altered clotting; maladaptive stress response; neuro-sensory alteration. *Minor:* Chilling; perspiring; dyspnea; cough; itching; restlessness; insomnia; fatigue; anorexia; weakness; immobility; disorientation; pressure sores.

SELF-CARE DEFICIT(S): ADL See ACTIVITY INTOLERANCE; also see SELF-CARE DEFICIT(S) which follow. Other diagnoses may also be applicable to individual circumstances.

SELF-CARE DEFICIT(S) A state in which the individual experiences an impaired ability to perform or complete one or more of the following activities for oneself:
BATHING/HYGIENE: Defining Characteristics: Inability to wash body or body parts; inability* to obtain or get to water source; inability to regulate temperature or flow.
DRESSING/GROOMING: Defining Characteristics: Impaired ability to put on or take off necessary items of clothing; impaired ability to obtain or replace articles of clothing; impaired ability to fasten clothing; inability to maintain appearance at a satisfactory level.
FEEDING: Defining Characteristics: Inability to bring food from a receptacle to one's mouth.
TOILETING: **Defining Characteristics:**

Unable to get to toilet or commode; unable to sit on or rise from toilet or commode; unable to manipulate clothing for toileting; unable to carry out proper toilet hygiene; unable to flush toilet or commode. Note: See *Suggested Functional Level Classification* under diagnosis MOBILITY, IMPAIRED PHYSICAL.

SELF-ESTEEM DISTURBANCE
Negative self-evaluation of capabilities, or negative feelings about self or own capabilities, which may be directly or indirectly expressed. **Defining Characteristics:** Self-negating verbalizations; expressions of shame/guilt; evaluates self as unable to deal with events; rationalizes away/rejects positive feedback and exaggerates negative feedback about self; hesitant to try new things/situations; denial of problems obvious to others; projection of blame/responsibility for problems; rationalizing personal failures; hypersensitive to slight or criticism; grandiosity.

SENSORY/PERCEPTUAL ALTERATIONS: VISUAL, AUDITORY, KINESTHETIC, GUSTATORY, TACTILE, OLFACTORY (SPECIFY) A state in which an individual experiences a change in the amount or patterning of oncoming stimuli accompanied by a diminished, exaggerated, distorted, or impaired response to such stimuli. **Defining Characteristics:** Disoriented in time, in place, or with persons; altered abstraction; altered conceptualization; change in problem-solving abilities; reported or measured change in sensory acuity; change in behavior pattern; anxiety; apathy; change in usual response to stimuli; indication of body-image alteration; restlessness; irritability; altered communication patterns. **Other Possible Characteristics:** Complaints of fatigue; alteration in posture; change in muscular tension; inappropriate responses; hallucinations.

SEXUALITY PATTERNS, ALTERED The state in which an individual expresses concern regarding his/her sexuality. **Defining Characteristics:** Reported difficulties, limitations, or changes in sexual behaviors or activities.

SKIN INTEGRITY, IMPAIRED A state in which the individual's skin is adversely altered. **Defining Characteristics:**

Disruption of skin surface; destruction of skin layers; invasion of body structures.

SKIN INTEGRITY, IMPAIRED: HIGH RISK FOR A state in which the individual's skin is at risk of being adversely altered. **Defining Characteristics:** *Presence of risk factors such as: External (environmental):* Hypo- or hyperthermia; chemical substance; mechanical factors (shearing forces, pressure, restraint); radiation; physical immobilization; excretions/secretions; humidity. *Internal (somatic):* Medication; alterations in nutritional state (obesity, emaciation); altered metabolic state; altered circulation; altered sensation; altered pigmentation; skeletal prominence; developmental factors; alterations in skin turgor (change in elasticity); psychogenic; immunologic.

SLEEP PATTERN DISTURBANCE A state in which disruption of sleep time causes discomfort or interferes with desired lifestyle. **Defining Characteristics:** Verbal complaints of difficulty falling asleep; awakening earlier or later than desired; interrupted sleep; verbal complaints of not feeling well-rested; changes in behavior and performance (increasing irritability, restlessness, disorientation, lethargy, listlessness); physical signs (mild fleeting nystagmus, slight hand tremor, ptosis of eyelid, expressionless face, dark circles under eyes, frequent yawning, changes in posture); thick speech with mispronunciation and incorrect words.

SWALLOWING, IMPAIRED The state in which an individual has decreased ability to voluntarily pass fluids and/or solids from the mouth to the stomach. **Defining Characteristics:** *Major:* Observed evidence of difficulty in swallowing, e.g., stasis of food in oral cavity, coughing/choking. *Minor:* Evidence of aspiration.

THERAPEUTIC REGIMEN MANAGEMENT (INDIVIDUALS), INEFFECTIVE A pattern of regulating and integrating into daily living a program for treatment of illness and the sequelae of illness that is unsatisfactory for meeting specific health goals. **Defining Characteristics:** *Major:* Choices of daily living ineffective for meeting the goals of a treatment or prevention program. *Minor:* Acceleration (expected or unexpected) of illness symptoms; verbalized desire to manage the treatment of illness and prevention of sequelae; verbalized difficulty with regulation/integration of one or more prescribed regimens for treatment of illness and its effects or prevention of complications; verbalized that did not take action to include treatment regimens in daily routines; verbalized that did not take action to reduce risk factors for progression of illness and sequelae.

THOUGHT PROCESSES, ALTERED A state in which an individual experiences a disruption in cognitive operations and activities. **Defining Characteristics:** Accurate interpretation of environment; cognitive dissonance; distractibility; memory deficit/problems; egocentricity; hyper- or hypovigilance. **Other Possible Characteristics:** Inappropriate or non-reality-based thinking.

TISSUE INTEGRITY, IMPAIRED A state in which an individual experiences damage to mucous membrane, corneal, integumentary, or subcutaneous tissue. **Defining Characteristics:** Damaged or destroyed tissue (cornea, mucous membrane, integumentary, or subcutaneous).

TISSUE PERFUSION, ALTERED: RENAL, CEREBRAL, CARDIOPULMONARY, GASTROINTESTINAL, PERIPHERAL (SPECIFY TYPE) The state in which an individual experiences a decrease in nutrition and oxygenation at the cellular level due to a deficit in capillary blood supply. **Defining Characteristics:** Skin temperature: cold in extremities. Skin color: dependent, blue or purple and pale on elevation; color does not return on lowering of leg; diminished arterial pulsations. Skin quality: shining; lack of lanugo; slow healing of lesions; gangrene; slow-growing, dry, brittle nails. **Other Possible Characteristics:** Claudication; blood pressure changes in extremities; bruits.

TOTAL INCONTINENCE See URINARY INCONTINENCE, TOTAL and BOWEL INCONTINENCE.

URINARY ELIMINATION, ALTERED The state in which the individual experiences a disturbance in urine elimination. **Defining Characteristics:** Dysuria; frequency; hesitancy; incontinence; nocturia; retention; urgency.

URINARY INCONTINENCE, TOTAL The state in which an individual experiences a continuous and unpredictable loss of urine. **Defining Characteristics:** *Major:* Constant flow of urine occurs at unpredictable times without distention or uninhibited bladder contractions/spasm; unsuccessful incontinence refractory treatments; nocturia. *Minor:* Lack of perineal or bladder filling awareness; unawareness of incontinence.

URINARY RETENTION The state in which the individual experiences incomplete emptying of the bladder. **Defining Characteristics:** *Major:* Bladder distention; small, frequent voiding or absence of urine output. *Minor:* Sensation of bladder fullness; dribbling; residual urine; dysuria; overflow incontinence.

VENTILATION, SPONTANEOUS: INABILITY TO SUSTAIN A state in which the response pattern of decreased energy reserves results in an individual's inability to maintain breathing adequate to support. **Defining Characteristics:** *Major:* Dyspnea; increased metabolic rate. *Minor:* Increased restlessness; apprehension; increased use of accessory muscles; decreased tidal volume; increased heart rate; decreased PO_2; increased PCO_2; decreased cooperation; decreased SaO_2.

Ackerman, M. H.: "The Effect of Saline Lavage Prior to Suctioning," *American Journal of Critical Care, 2(4)*, 1993, pp. 326-330.

Ackley, B., and G. Ladwig: *Nursing Diagnosis Handbook: A Guide to Planning Care*, Mosby Year Book, St. Louis, 1993.

Alberti, K. G. M. M., R. A. DeFronzo, H. Keen, and P. Zimmet: *International Textbook of Diabetes Mellitus*, II, John Wiley & Sons, New York, 1992.

Arthritis Foundation: *Systemic Lupus Erythematosis*, Arthritis Foundation of Georgia, 1990.

Axton, Sharon E., and Terry Fugate: *Neonatal and Pediatric Critical Care Plans*, Williams and Wilkins Publishing Company, Baltimore, 1989.

_____ : *Pediatric Care Plans*, Addison-Wesley Nursing, Redwood City, Calif., 1993.

Baler, H., R. Begin, and M. Sackner: "Effect of Airway Diameter, Suction Catheters, and the Bronchofiberscope on Airflow in Endotracheal and Tracheostomy Tubes," *Heart and Lung, 5(2)*, 1976, pp. 235-238.

Barkin, R.: *Pediatric Emergency Medicine: Concepts and Clinical Practice*, Mosby Year Book, St. Louis, 1992.

Bayne, Marilyn Varner, and Donna D. Iqnatavicus: *Medical-Surgical Nursing: A Nursing Process Approach*, W. B. Saunders Company, Philadelphia, 1991.

Behrman, Richard E., Robert M. Kliegman, Waldo E. Nelson, and Victor C. Vaughan III: *Nelson Textbook of Pediatrics*, 14th ed., W. B. Saunders Company, Philadelphia, 1992.

Berkow, R., and A. Fletcher: *The Merck Manual*, 15th ed., Merck Sharp and Dohme International Laboratories, N.J., 1987.

Bernard, M., M. Chard, J. Howe, and G. Scipien: *Pediatric Nursing Care*, Mosby Year Book, St. Louis, 1990.

Betz, C. L., and E. C. Poster: *Mosby's Pediatric Nursing Reference*, 2d ed., Mosby Year Book, St. Louis, 1992.

Brunner, L., and D. Suddarth: *The Lippincott Manual of Nursing Practice*, 4th ed., J. B. Lippincott Company, Philadelphia, 1986.

_____ : *Textbook of Medical-Surgical Nursing*, 6th ed., J. B. Lippincott Company, Philadelphia, 1988.

Burgess, M. C.: "Initial Management of a Patient With Extensive Burn Injury," *Critical Care Nursing Clinics of North America, 3(2)*, 1991, pp. 165-179.

Campbell, V., E. Chipps, and N. Clarin: *Neurologic Disorders*, Mosby Year Book, St. Louis, 1992.

Carpenito, Lynda Juall: *Handbook of Nursing Diagnosis*, J. B. Lippincott Company, Philadelphia, 1989.

_____ : *Handbook of Nursing Diagnosis*, J. B. Lippincott Company, Philadelphia, 1991.

_____ : *Handbook of Nursing Diagnosis*, 5th ed., J. B. Lippincott Company, Philadelphia, 1993.

_____ : *Nursing Diagnosis: Application to Clinical Practice*, 3rd ed., J. B. Lippincott Company, Philadelphia, 1989.

_____ : *Nursing Diagnosis: Application to Clinical Practice*, 5th ed., J. B. Lippincott Company, Philadelphia, 1993.

Carroll-Johnson, Rose Mary (Ed.): *North American Nursing Diagnosis Association Classification of Nursing Diagnoses: Proceedings of the Ninth Conference*, J.B. Lippincott Company, Philadelphia, 1991.

Cassmeyer, Virginia, Barbara C. Long, Wilma Phipps, and Nancy Woods: *Medical-Surgical Nursing: Concepts and Clinical Practice*, Mosby Year Book, St. Louis, 1991.

Castiglia, P. T., and R. E. Harbin: *Child Health Care*, J. B. Lippincott Company, Philadelphia, 1992.

Chulay, M., and G. M. Graeber: "Efficacy of Hyperinflation and Hyper-oxygenation Suctioning Intervention," *Heart and Lung, 17(1)*, 1988, pp. 15-22.

Cohen, F., and J. Durham: *Women, Children, and HIV / AIDS*, Springer Publishing Company, New York, 1993.

Cox, H., M. Hinz, M. S. Lubano, S. Newfield, N. Rindenour, M. Slater, and K. Sridaromont: *Clinical Application of Nursing Diagnosis: Adult, Child, Women's, Psychiatric, Terontic and Home Health Considerations*, 2d ed., F. A. Davis Company, Philadelphia, 1993.

Denson, Cynthia, and William Terry: "Hypospadias Repair," *AORN Journal*, April 1988, pp. 906-924.

DeVita, V., S. Hellman, and S. Rosenberg: *Principles and Practice of Oncology*, J. B. Lippincott Company, Philadelphia, 1993.

Doenges, M. S., and M. F. Moorhouse: *Nurses' Pocket Guide: Nursing Diagnoses with Interventions*, F. A. Davis Company, Philadelphia, 1993.

Duncan, D. J., and D. M. Driscoll: "Burn Wound Management," *Critical Care Nursing Clinics of North America, 3(2)*, 1992, pp. 199-219.

Edelman, C. L., and C. L. Mandle: *Health Promotion Throughout the Lifespan*, Mosby Year Book, St. Louis, 1990.

Engstrom, I.: "Family Interaction and Locus of Control in Children and Adolescents with Inflammatory Bowel Disease," *Journal of the American Academy of Child and Adolescent Psychiatry*, November 1991, pp. 913-920.

_____ : "Parental Distress and Social interaction in Families with Children With Inflammatory Bowel Disease," *Journal of the American Academy of Child and Adolescent Psychiatry*, November 1991, pp. 904-912.

Flaskerud, J.: *AIDS / HIV Infections: A Reference Guide for Nursing Professionals*, W. B. Saunders Company, Philadelphia, 1989.

Flynn, J. P., and E. A. Mahoney: *Handbook of Surgical Nursing*, Fleschner Publishing Company, New Haven, Conn., 1983.

Foley, G. V., D. Fochtman, and K. H. Mooney: *Nursing Care of the Child with Cancer*, W. B. Saunders Company, Philadelphia, 1993.

Foster, R., M. Hunsburger, and J. Anderson: *Family-Centered Nursing Care of Children*, W. B. Saunders Company, Philadelphia, 1989.

Gordon, Marjory: *Manual of Nursing Diagnosis, 1993-1994*, Mosby Year Book, St. Louis, 1993.

Grartside, Gretta: "Fit for Nursing: The Ultimate Rebellion," *Nursing Times*, May 1989, p. 50.

Greenberg, Cindy Smith (Ed.): *Nursing Care Planning Guidelines for Children*, Williams and Wilkins Publishing Company, Baltimore, 1989.

Gulanick, Meg R., Michele Knoll Puzas, and Cynthia R. Wilson: *Nursing Care Plans for Newborns and Children: Acute and Critical Care*, Mosby Year Book, St. Louis, 1992.

Guyton, Arthur C.: *Textbook of Medical Physiology*, W. B. Saunders Company, Philadelphia, 1991.

Hagenah, G. C., J. F. Harrigan, and M. Campbell: "Inflammatory Bowel Disease in Children," *Nursing Clinics of North America*, March 1984, pp. 27-39.

Haire-Joshu, Debra: *Management of Diabetes Mellitus*, Mosby Year Book, St. Louis, 1990.

Hazinski, Mary Fran: *Nursing Care of the Critically Ill Child*, C.V. Mosby, St. Louis, 1984.

_____ : *Nursing Care of the Critically Ill Child*, 2nd ed., Mosby Year Book, Philadelphia, 1992.

BIBLIOGRAPHY

Hirsh, J., M. McFarland, June Thompson, and Susan Tucker: *Mosby's Clinical Nursing*, Mosby Year Book, St. Louis, 1993.

Holbrook, P.: *Textbook of Pediatric Critical Care*, W. B. Saunders Company, Philadelphia, 1993.

Holloway, Nancy M.: *Critical-care Care Plans*, Springhouse Corporation, Springhouse, Pa., 1989.

Horton, Hilda, Pat Crutchfield, and Connie Garrison: "Hypospadias: When Baby Boys Need Surgery," *RN*, June 1990, pp. 48-52.

Huddleston, K., and A. Ferraro: "Preparing Families of Children with Gastrostomies," *Pediatric Nursing, 17(2)*, 1991, pp. 153-158.

_____ and K. Palmer: "A Button for Gastrostomy Feedings," *MCN, 15*, 1990, pp. 315-319.

Ibrahim, K.: "Overview of Childhood Fractures," *Pediatric Nursing, 10*, 1984, pp. 57-65.

Jackson, Debra Broadwell, and Rebecca B. Saunders: *Child Health Nursing: A Comprehensive Approach to the Care of Children and Their Families*, J. B. Lippincott Company, Philadelphia, 1993.

Jackson, Deirdre F.: "Nursing Care Plan: Home Management of Children With BPD," *Pediatric Nursing*, September-October 1986, pp. 342-348.

Jaffe, Marie S.: *Medical-Surgical Nursing Care Plans*, Appleton and Lange Publishers, Hartford, Conn., 1992.

_____: *Pediatric Nursing Care Plans*, Skidmore-Roth Publishers, El Paso, Tex., 1993.

James, S., and S. Mott: *Child Health Nursing: Essential Care of Children and Families*, Addison-Wesley Publishing Company, Reading, Mass., 1988.

Johnson, D. G.: "Current Thinking on the Role of Surgery in Gastroesophageal Reflux," in T. E. Lobe and M. Schwartz (Eds.), *The Pediatric Clinics of North America, 32(5)*, 1985, pp. 1165-1170.

Johnson, Suzanne Hall: *Nursing Assessment and Strategies for the Family at Risk*, J. B. Lippincott Company, Philadelphia, 1986.

Jung, R. C., and L. S. Gottlieb: "Comparison of Tracheobronchial Suction Catheters in Humans," *Chest, 69(2)*, 1976, pp. 179-181.

Kelley, Mary Ann, *Nursing Diagnosis Source Book: Guidelines for Clinical Applications*, Appleton-Century-Crofts, Norwalk, Conn., 1985.

Kennelly, C.: "Tracheostomy Care: Parents As Learners," *MCN, 12(4)*, 1987, pp. 264-267.

Kenner, Carole, Ann Brueggemeyer, and Laurie P. Gunderson: *Comprehensive Neonatal Nursing: A Physiologic Perspective*, W. B. Saunders Company, Philadelphia, 1993.

Kenney, M.: "Hospital to Home: Care of the Child with a Tracheostomy," *Neonatal Network*, August 1987, pp. 21-24.

Kim, Mi Ja, Gertrude K. McFarland, and Audrey M. McLane: *Pocket Guide to Nursing Diagnoses*, 5th ed., Mosby Year Book, St. Louis, 1993.

Klaus, M. H., and A. A. Fanaroff: *Care of the High-risk Neonate*, W. B. Saunders Company, Philadelphia, 1993.

Kleiber, C., N. Krutzfield, and E. Rose: "Acute Histologic Changes in the Tracheobronchial Tree Associated with Different Suction Catheter Insertion Techniques," *Heart and Lung, 17(1)*, 1988, pp. 10-14.

Kleinman, R. E., W. E. Balistreri, M. B. Heyman, B. S. Kirschner, A. M. Lake, K. J. Motil, E. Seidman, and J. N. Udall, Jr.: "Nutritional Support for Pediatric Patients with Inflammatory Bowel Disease," *Journal of Pediatric Gastroenterology and Nutrition*, January 1989, pp. 812.

Knuppel, R. A., and J. E. Drukker: *High-risk Pregnancy: A Team Approach*, 2d ed., W. B. Saunders Company, Philadelphia, 1993.

Kravitz, Melva (Ed.): *AACN Clinical Issues in Critical Care Nursing: Burn Care*, J. B. Lippincott Company, Philadelphia, 1993.

LeBlanc, K. B., and F. E. Foustell: "Assessment of the Neonatal Respiratory System," *AACN Clinical Issues in Critical Care Nursing, 1(2)*, 1990, pp. 401-408.

Lebovitz, Harold: *Therapy for Diabetes Mellitus and Related Disorders*, American Diabetes Association, Alexandria, Va., 1991.

Lederer, J., G. Marculescu, B. Mosnik, and N. Seaby, *Care Planning Pocket Guide: A Nursing Diagnosis Approach*, Addison-Wesley, Redwood City, Calif., 1991.

Leuner, J. D., A. K. Manton, D. B. Kelliher, S. P. Sullivan, and M. Doherty: *Mastering the Nursing Process: A Case Method Approach*, F. A. Davis Company, Philadelphia, 1990.

Levy, J.: *Practical Approaches to Pediatric Gastroenterology*, Year Book Medical, Chicago, 1988.

Link, W. J., E. E. Spaeth, W. M. Wahle, W. Penny, and J.L. Glover: "The Influence

of Suction Catheter Tip Design on Tracheobronchial Trauma and Fluid Tip Aspiration," *Anesthesia and Analgesia, 55(2)*, 1976, pp. 290-297.

Lomholt, N.: "Design and Function of Tracheal Suction Catheters," *ACTA Anaesthesia Scandinavia, 26*, 1982, pp. 13.

Long, Barbara C., and Wilma Phipps: *Essentials of Medical- Surgical Nursing*, C.V. Mosby, St. Louis, 1985.

Lupus Foundation of America: *Kidney Involvement in Lupus*, The Lupus Foundation, Columbus, Ohio, 1992.

Marlow, D., and B. Redding: *Textbook of Pediatric Nursing*, W. B. Saunders Company, Philadelphia, 1988.

Mattson, Susan., and Judy E. Smith: *Core Curriculum for Maternal-Newborn Nursing*, W. B. Saunders Company, Philadelphia, 1993.

Mayers, Marlene: *Clinical Care Plans: Pediatric Nursing*, Markham-McKenzie Publishers, Eugene, Oreg., 1991.

_____: *Clinical Care Plans: Perinatal Nursing*, Markham- McKenzie Publishers, Eugene, Oreg., 1991.

_____: *Clinical Care Plans: Medical Nursing*, Markham-McKenzie Publishers, Eugene, Oreg., 1989.

_____: *Clinical Care Plans: Orthopedic and Neurologic Nursing*, Markham-McKenzie Publishers, Eugene, Oreg., 1989.

_____: *Clinical Care Plans: Surgical Nursing*, Markham-McKenzie Publishers, Eugene, Oreg., 1989.

McCloskey, J. C., and G. M. Bulechek: *Nursing Interventions Classification (NIC)*, Mosby Year Book, St. Louis, 1992.

McCulloch, F. L., and L. M. Evans: "Assessment of Neurovascular Status in Children," *Orthopedic Nursing, 4*, 1985, pp. 19-25.

McFarland, G., and E. McFarland: *Nursing Diagnosis and Intervention: Planning for Patient Care*, 2d ed., Mosby Year Book, St. Louis, 1993.

Meades, Stephen: "Suggested Community Psychiatric Nursing Interventions with Clients Suffering from Anorexia Nervosa and Bulimia Nervosa," *Journal of Advanced Nursing*, March 1993, pp. 364-370.

Meeker, M. H., and J. C. Rothrock: *Alexander's Care of the Patient in Surgery*, Mosby Year Book, St. Louis, 1991.

Meize-Grochowski, A. T.: "When the Dx is Crohn's Disease," *RN*, February 1991, pp. 52-56.

Merenstein, G., and S. Gardner: *Handbook of Neonatal Intensive Care*, 2d ed., C.V. Mosby, St. Louis, 1989.

Mott, S., S. James, and A. Sperhac: *Nursing Care of Children and Families*, 2d ed., Addison-Wesley Nursing, Redwood City, Calif., 1990.

Neiman, G., and J. Lehman: *A Parents' Guide: Cleft Lip and Palate and Other Craniofacial Problems*, Plastic and Reconstructive Surgeons Incorporated, 1990.

Nelson, Nancy P., and Julie Beckel (Eds.): *Nursing Care Plans for the Pediatric Patient*, C.V. Mosby, St. Louis, 1987. and : *Nursing Care Plans for the Pediatric Patient*, C.V. Mosby, St. Louis, 1990.

Newberger, Eli H.: *Child Abuse*, Little, Brown, and Company, Boston, 1982.

Newman, J., and G. Scott: *Pediatric Nursing*, Springhouse Corporation, Springhouse, Pa., 1990.

North American Nursing Diagnosis Association: *NANDA Nursing Diagnoses: Definitions and Classifications 1992 – 1993,* North American Nursing Diagnosis Association, Philadelphia, 1992.

Nufer, Nancy: "Pediatric Management Problems," *Pediatric Nursing*, July-August 1989, pp. 388-389.

Nugent, Jan (Ed.): *Acute Respiratory Care of the Neonate*, NICU Incorporated, Petaluma, Calif., 1991.

Osenges, M., Alice Neissler, and Mary Francis Moorehouse: *Nursing Care Plans: Guidelines for Planning and Documenting Care*, F. A. Davis Company, Philadelphia, 1993.

Pillitteri, Adele: *Maternal and Child Health Nursing: Care of the Childbearing and Childrearing Family*, J. B. Lippincott Company, Philadelphia, 1992.

Platzker, Arnold C. G.: "Chronic Lung Disease of Infancy," in Roberta A. Ballard (Ed.), *Pediatric Care of the ICN Graduate*, W. B. Saunders Company, Philadelphia, 1988.

Rand-Doxzon, Mindy, Carol Vest, and Lois Linden (Eds.): "Collaborative Problem #8: Croup, Laryngotracheobronchitis, Epiglottitis," in *Clinical Practice Guidelines*, Children's Hospital, Omaha, Neb., 1992.

Regan, M.: "Tracheal Mucosal Injury: The Nurse's Role," *Nursing (London), 29*, 1988, pp. 1064-1066.

Reiner, Anne: *Manual of Patient Care Standards*, Aspen Publishers, Gaithersburg, Va., 1993.

"Report of the Second Task Force on Blood Pressure Control in Children," *Pediatrics, 79(1)*, 1987, pp. 1-25.

Ross, R., R. Bolinger, and W. Pinsky: "Grading the Severity of Congestive Heart Failure in Infants," *Pediatric Cardiology*, April 1992, pp. 72-75.

Saint Louis Children's Hospital Standard Plan of Care as Defined in Data Base as of 09 / 01 / 93, Saint Louis Children's Hospital, St. Louis, 1993.

Sitton, Ellen: "Early and Late Radiation-Induced Skin Alterations, Part II: Nursing Care of Irradiated Skin," *Oncology Nursing Forum, 19(6)*, 1992, pp. 907- 912.

Smeltzer, S., and B. Bare: *Brunner and Suddarth's Textbook of Medical Surgical Nursing*, 7th ed., J. B. Lippincott Company, Philadelphia, 1992.

Sparacino, L. L.: "Psychosocial Considerations for the Adolescent and Young Adult with Inflammatory Bowel Disease," *Nursing Clinics of North America*, March 1984, pp. 41-49.

Sparks, Shelia M., and Cynthia M. Taylor: *Nursing Diagnosis Reference Manual: An Indispensable Guide to Better Patient Care*, Springhouse Corporation, Springhouse, Pa., 1991.

Speer, Kathleen Morgan: *Pediatric Care Plans*, Springhouse Corporation, Springhouse, Pa., 1990.

Station 3 Clinical Standards Council: *Standard of Care for the Child Receiving Chemotherapy*, Minneapolis Children's Medical Center Nursing Division, Minneapolis, January 1991.

_____ : *Standard of Care for the Child with Neutropenia*, Minneapolis Children's Medical Center Nursing Division, Minneapolis, September 1990.

_____ : *Standard of Care for the Child with Newly Diagnosed Leukemia*, Minneapolis Children's Medical Center Nursing Division, Minneapolis, 1991.

Stotts, N. A., K. A. Fitzgerald, and K. R. Williams: "Care of the Patient Critically Ill with Inflammatory Bowel Disease," *Nursing Clinics of North America*, March 1984, pp. 61-69.

Suddarth, Doris Smith: *The Lippincott Manual of Nursing Practice*, 5th ed., J. B. Lippincott Company, Philadelphia, 1991.

Swartz, S. I., and H. Ellis: *Mangot's Abdominal Operations, 1*, 8th ed., Appleton-Century-Crofts, Norwalk, Conn., 1985.

Tachdjean, Mihran O.: *Pediatric Orthopedics, 2*, W. B. Saunders Company, Philadelphia, 1990.

Task Force on Pediatric AIDS: "Pediatric Guidelines for Infection Control of Human Immunodeficiency Virus (Acquired Immunodeficiency Virus) in Hospitals, Medical Offices, Schools and Other Settings," *Pediatrics 82(5)*, 1988.

Texas Children's Hospital, *Nursing Standard of Patient Care*, Texas Children's Hospital, Houston, 1992.

Tucker, S. M., M. Breeding, M. M. Canobbio, G. Jacquet, E. V. Paquette, M. F. Wells, and M. Williams: *Patient Care Standards*, Mosby Year Book, St. Louis, 1975.

Tucker, S. M., M. M. Canobbio, E. V. Paquette, M. F. Wells, and M. Williams: *Patient Care Standards: Nursing Process, Diagnosis, and Outcome*, Mosby Year Book, St. Louis, 1988.

Ulrich, S., S. Canale, and S. Wendell: *Nursing Care Planning Guides: A Nursing Diagnosis Approach*, 2d ed., W. B. Saunders Company, Philadelphia, 1990.

Waterhouse, Lorraine: *Child Abuse and Child Abusers: Protection and Prevention*, Jessica Kingsley Publishers, Philadelphia, 1993.

Weimer, William, *Emergent and Urgent Neurology*, J. B. Lippincott Company, Philadelphia, 1992.

Wesorick, Bonnie: *Standards of Nursing Care: A Model for Clinical Practice*, J. B. Lippincott Company, Philadelphia, 1990.

Whaley, Lucille F., and Donna L. Wong: *Essentials of Pediatric Nursing*, 4th ed., C.V. Mosby, Philadephia, 1993.

_____ and _____ : *Nursing Care of Infants and Children*, 3rd ed., C.V. Mosby, St. Louis, 1987.

_____ and _____ : *Nursing Care of Infants and Children*, 4th ed., Mosby Year Book, St. Louis, 1991.

Wong, Donna L., and Lucille F. Whaley: *Clinical Manual of Pediatric Nursing*, C.V. Mosby, St. Louis, 1986.

_____ and _____ : *Clinical Manual of Pediatric Nursing*, 3d ed., Mosby Year Book, St. Louis, 1990.

Yogev, R., and E. Conner: *Management of HIV Infection in Infants and Children*, Mosby Year Book, St. Louis, 1992.

Zink, M.: "Biliary Atresia: Nursing Diagnosis and Management," *Journal of Enterostomal Therapy, 12*, 1985, pp. 128-139.

INDEX